Fibromyalgia, Chronic Fatigue Syndrome, and Repetitive Strain Injury

Current Concepts in Diagnosis, Management, Disability, and Health Economics

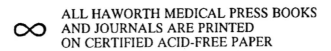

ALL HAWORTH MEDICAL PRESS BOOKS
AND JOURNALS ARE PRINTED
ON CERTIFIED ACID-FREE PAPER

Fibromyalgia, Chronic Fatigue Syndrome, and Repetitive Strain Injury

Current Concepts in Diagnosis, Management, Disability, and Health Economics

Andrew Chalmers, MD
Geoffrey Owen Littlejohn, MD
Irving Salit, MD
Frederick Wolfe, MD
Editors

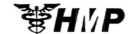

The Haworth Medical Press
An Imprint of
The Haworth Press, Inc.
New York · London

6 16. 74
F443

Published by

The Haworth Medical Press, 10 Alice Street, Binghamton, NY 13904-1580 USA

The Haworth Medical Press is an imprint of The Haworth Press, Inc., 10 Alice Street, Binghamton, NY 13904-1580 USA.

Fibromyalgia, Chronic Fatigue Syndrome, and Repetitive Strain Injury: Current Concepts in Diagnosis, Management, Disability, and Health Economics has also been published as *Journal of Musculoskeletal Pain*, Volume 3, Number 2 1995.

© 1995 by The Haworth Press, Inc. All rights reserved. No part of this work may be reproduced or utilized in any form or by any means, electronic or mechanical, including photocopying, microfilm and recording, or by any information storage and retrieval system, without permission in writing from the publisher. Printed in the United States of America.

The development, preparation, and publication of this work has been undertaken with great care. However, the publisher, employees, editors, and agents of The Haworth Press and all imprints of The Haworth Press, Inc., including The Haworth Medical Press and Pharmaceutical Products Press, are not responsible for any errors contained herein or for consequences that may ensue from use of materials or information contained in this work. Opinions expressed by the author(s) are not necessarily those of The Haworth Press, Inc.

Library of Congress Cataloging-in-Publication Data

Fibromyalgia, chronic fatigue syndrome, and repetitive strain injury: current concepts in diagnosis, management, disability, and health economics / Andrew Chalmers . . . [et al.], editors.
      p. cm.
      (Journal of musculoskeletal pain; v. 3, no. 2)
      "A compilation of papers presented at the Physical Medicine Research Foundation's 8th International Symposium"–Introd.
      "Has also been published as Journal of musculoskeletal pain, volume 3, number 2, 1995"–T.p. verso.
      Includes bibliographical references and index.
      ISBN 1-56024-744-4 (alk. paper)
      1. Fibromyalgia–Congresses. 2. Myofascial pain syndromes–Congresses. 3. Chronic fatigue syndrome–Congresses. 4. Overuse injuries–Congresses. I. Chalmers, Andrew. II. Physical Medicine Research Foundation. International Symposium. (8th: 1994: University of British Columbia) III. Series.
      [DNLM: 1. Fibromyalgia–congresses. 2. Fatigue Syndrome, Chronic–congresses. 3. Repetition Strain Injury–congresses. W1 J0775RK v.3 no.2 1995 / WE 544 F4415 1995]
RC927.3.F52 1995
616.7–dc20
DNLM/DLC
for Library of Congress

95-30842
CIP

ALLEN COUNTY COMMUNITY
COLLEGE LIBRARY
Iola, Kansas 66749

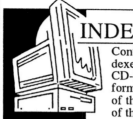

INDEXING & ABSTRACTING

Contributions to this publication are selectively indexed or abstracted in print, electronic, online, or CD-ROM version[s] of the reference tools and information services listed below. This list is current as of the copyright date of this publication. See the end of this section for additional notes.

- *Behavioral Medicine Abstracts,* Pain Evaluation and Treatment Institute, 4601 Baum Boulevard, Pittsburgh, PA 15213-1217

- *Cambridge Scientific Abstracts,* Health & Safety Science Abstracts, Cambridge Information Group, 7200 Wisconsin Avenue #601, Bethesda, MD 20814

- *Dental Abstracts,* Mosby-Year Book, Inc., 200 N. LaSalle Street, Chicago, IL 60601-1080

- *Ergonomics Abstracts,* Taylor & Francis, Ltd., Rankine Road, Basingstoke, Hants RG24 0PR, England

- *Excerpta Medica/Electronic Publishing Division,* Elsevier Science Inc., Secondary Publishing Division, 655 Avenue of the Americas, New York, NY 10010

- *INTERNET ACCESS [& additional networks] Bulletin Board for Libraries ["BUBL"], coverage of information resources on INTERNET, JANET, and other networks.*
  - JANET X.29: UK.AC.BATH.BUBL or 00006012101300
  - TELNET: BUBL.BATH.AC.UK or 138.38.32.45 login 'bubl'
  - Gopher: BUBL.BATH.AC.UK [138.32.32.45]. Port 7070
  - World Wide Web: http://www.bubl.bath.ac.uk./BUBL/home.html
  - NISSWAIS: telnetniss.ac.uk [for the NISS gateway]
  The Andersonian Library, Curran Building, 101 St. James Road, Glasgow G4 ONS, Scotland

- *Pharmacist's Letter "Abstracts Section,"* Therapeutic Research Center, 8834 Hildreth Lane, Stockton, CA 95212

- *Physical Therapy "Abstracts Section,"* American Physical Therapy Association, 1111 North Fairfax Street, Alexandria, VA 22314-1488

[continued]

56838

- *Referativnyi Zhurnal [Abstracts Journal of the Institute of Scientific Information of the Republic of Russia],* The Institute of Scientific Information, Baltijskaja ul., 14, Moscow A-219, Republic of Russia

- *SilverPlatter Information, Inc. "CD-ROM/online,"* Information Resources Group, P.O. Box 50550, Pasadena, CA 91115-0550

- *Sport Database/Discus,* Sport Information Resource Center, 1600 James Naismith Drive, Suite 107, Gloucester, Ontario K1B 5N4, Canada

---

SPECIAL BIBLIOGRAPHIC NOTES

*related to special Journal issues [separates]
and indexing/abstracting*

☐ indexing/abstracting services in this list will also cover material in any "separate" that is co-published simultaneously with Haworth's special thematic journal issue or DocuSerial. Indexing/abstracting usually covers material at the article/chapter level.

☐ monographic co-editions are intended for either non-subscribers or libraries which intend to purchase a second copy for their circulating collections.

☐ monographic co-editions are reported to all jobbers/wholesalers/approval plans. The source journal is listed as the "series" to assist the prevention of duplicate purchasing in the same manner utilized for books-in-series.

☐ to facilitate user/access services all indexing/abstracting services are encouraged to utilize the co-indexing entry note indicated at the bottom of the first page of each article/chapter/contribution.

☐ this is intended to assist a library user of any reference tool [whether print, electronic, online, or CD-ROM] to locate the monographic version if the library has purchased this version but not a subscription to the source journal.

☐ individual articles/chapters in any Haworth publication are also available through the Haworth Document Delivery Services [HDDS].

Fibromyalgia, Chronic Fatigue Syndrome, and Repetitive Strain Injury

Current Concepts in Diagnosis, Management, Disability, and Health Economics

CONTENTS

Preface:
The Vancouver Conference

The proceedings which follow provide a summary of a conference on chronic fatigue syndrome [CFS], fibromyalgia syndrome [FS], and related disorders held in June, 1994, on the beautiful campus of the University of British Columbia, Vancouver, BC, Canada. The conference planner and host was Dr. Andrew Chalmers, Associate Professor of Medicine and Rheumatology and Associate Dean Undergraduate, University of British Columbia.

Many of the investigators known to be actively involved in the study of the target disorders were invited to present their viewpoints and later participate in discussions aimed at achieving a consensus. Contributors came from far flung points of the globe including England, Australia, the United States and Canada. In addition to the health professionals, the participants included representatives from the legal profession and the insurance industry of Canada.

The unique feature of this conference was to be its emphasis on disability and compensation. The importance of those issues was so substantial and opinions have traditionally varied so widely that there was much speculation about how the conference would proceed, what its outcome might be, and whether consensus really could be achieved on such divisive topics. There were also differing opinions regarding the relative merits of involving the insurance industry as both participants and sponsors of debates on questions which so clearly affected their services and profit margins. On the other hand, health care providers, and especially academic investigators, tend to be a rather independent lot and are not easily influenced to say or believe anything of which they are not convinced by the weight of the evidence.

[Haworth co-indexing entry note]: "Preface: The Vancouver Conference." Russell, I. Jon. Co-published simultaneously in the *Journal of Musculoskeletal Pain* (The Haworth Medical Press, an imprint of The Haworth Press, Inc.) Vol. 3, No. 2, 1995, pp. xv-xvi; and: *Fibromyalgia, Chronic Fatigue Syndrome, and Repetitive Strain Injury: Current Concepts in Diagnosis, Management, Disability, and Health Economics* (ed: Andrew Chalmers et al.) The Haworth Medical Press, an imprint of The Haworth Press, Inc., 1995, pp. xi-xii. Multiple copies of this article/chapter may be purchased from The Haworth Document Delivery Center [1-800-3-HAWORTH; 9:00 a.m. - 5:00 p.m. (EST)].

© 1995 by The Haworth Press, Inc. All rights reserved. *xi*

The format was 2 days of presentations to an audience composed of invited delegates and other registrants. Following the conclusion of the formal presentations, the delegates met intensively for several days to negotiate a comprehensive document of consensus. What follows in the pages of this issue are concise summaries of the formal presentations given during the first 2 days. The consensus document will be published elsewhere. In contrast to what might be expected, the consensus document does not necessarily mirror the information offered in the formal presentations.

Those who have been avid followers of trends in these fields will recognize an overall tenor in the manuscripts provided in this issue which differs subtly from the tones of previous conference proceedings. The impressions portrayed by the Minneapolis MYOPAIN conference in 1989 (1), the Copenhagen MYOPAIN conference in 1992 (2), and the NIH Fibromyalgia Workshop in 1993 (3) were that they focused respectively on a wide range of clinical features, on population epidemiology, and on biomedical pathogenesis. It is true that those meetings did some obeisance to psychological aspects of these conditions but, with the Vancouver conference, the pendulum seems to have perceptively swung back in the direction of viewing affective [psychological] pathology as a contributor to the underlying processes.

The reader is encouraged to follow closely the logic of each author's academic exercise, as he or she presents the arguments [concepts], pro and con, of the assigned topics. It can be reasonably anticipated that some of the presented hypotheses will be supported by future evidence while others may not. Notice also, how each presentation raises many more questions than it answers. This, of course, is the purpose of such interchange and the fruit of hearing different opinions. It now falls to each participant and reader to evaluate issues that have been raised, to embrace truth where it is found, to confront the unknown with a measure of confidence and to answer as many of the lingering questions as available methodology will allow.

I. Jon Russell, MD, PhD

REFERENCES

1. Fricton JR, Awad EA (editors): Advances in Pain Research and Therapy, Volume 17, Myofascial Pain and Fibromyalgia. Raven Press, New York, 1990.

2. Jacobsen S, Danneskiold-Samsoe B, Lund B (editors): Musculoskeletal Pain, Myofascial Pain Syndrome, and the Fibromyalgia Syndrome. Haworth Medical Press, Binghamton, NY, 1993.

3. Pillemer SR (editor): The Fibromyalgia Syndrome, Current Research and Future Directions in Epidemiology, Pathogenesis, and Treatment. Haworth Medical Press, Binghamton, NY, 1994.

Introduction:
The Physical Medicine Research Foundation's 8th International Symposium– Fibromyalgia, Chronic Fatigue Syndrome and Repetitive Strain Injury: Current Concepts in Diagnosis, Management and Cost Containment

Contained herein is a compilation of papers presented at the Physical Medicine Research Foundation's 8th International Symposium–Fibromyalgia, Chronic Fatigue Syndrome and Repetitive Strain Injury: Current Concepts in Diagnosis, Management and Cost Containment.

The symposium was sponsored by the Physical Medicine Research Foundation and the University of British Columbia. Chairs selected for their recognized international expertise in each of these areas [F. Wolfe, I. Salit, G. Littlejohn] provided names of individuals to present up-to-date information on each topic area.

The conference was designed to address etiology, pathogenesis, clinical features, treatment, disability, medico-legal issues and cost containment. The program agenda was issue-driven rather than condition-based, therefore the papers were presented in a manner which allowed delegates and speakers to see the overlap and differences between these conditions. The papers are in order of presentation.

[Haworth co-indexing entry note]: "Introduction: The Physical Medicine Research Foundation's 8th International Symposium–Fibromyalgia, Chronic Fatigue Syndrome and Repetitive Strain Injury: Current Concepts in Diagnosis, Management and Cost Containment." Chalmers, Andrew. Co-published simultaneously in the *Journal of Musculoskeletal Pain* (The Haworth Medical Press, an imprint of The Haworth Press, Inc.) Vol. 3, No. 2, 1995, pp. 1-2; and: *Fibromyalgia, Chronic Fatigue Syndrome, and Repetitive Strain Injury: Current Concepts in Diagnosis, Management, Disability, and Health Economics* (ed: Andrew Chalmers et al.) The Haworth Medical Press, an imprint of The Haworth Press, Inc., 1995, pp. 1-2. Multiple copies of this article/chapter may be purchased from The Haworth Document Delivery Center [1-800-3-HAWORTH; 9:00 a.m. - 5:00 p.m. (EST)].

© 1995 by The Haworth Press, Inc. All rights reserved.

1

Its purpose was to provide education for primary care physicians, specialist physicians, other health care disciplines, patients and the public. Presentations by patients were included, as well as opportunities for patients and the public to interact with the speakers.

A second purpose was to enable investigators in the three topic areas to come together and allow for cross-fertilization and an exchange of ideas that would hopefully inform future research and consensus in the particular areas focused on by the conference.

Following the symposium, a consensus conference was held to focus on fibromyalgia and chronic fatigue syndrome with particular emphasis on disability determination and medico-legal issues. The consensus documents will be published elsewhere.

The educational goal of the symposium appears to have been achieved for the majority of participants as measured by its ability to meet their perceived educational needs [overall rating 84%, perceived learning 78%].

Informal feedback from the speakers and consensus conference group suggest that the second goal of interchange between experts in the topic areas was also successful.

The ultimate success of the symposium will only be assessed in the future as agendas for future research unfold and clear understanding of these conditions allows for improved management and prevention of disability.

Acknowledgments: Section Chairs [F. Wolfe, I. Salit, G. Littlejohn], Local Planning Committee, Fibromyalgia Association of British Columbia, Myalgic Encephalomyelitis Society of BC, RSI project: Women and Work Educational Society and the Physical Medicine Research Foundation's Chronic Pain Support Group.

The symposium was supported by grants from: The Canadian Government [Health and Welfare Canada], The British Columbia Government [Ministry of Health], BC Tel Advanced Communications and Seaboard Life Insurance Co.

Andrew Chalmers, MD, FRCPC
Associate Professor of Medicine and Rheumatology
Associate Dean Undergraduate
University of British Columbia
3250-910 West 10th Avenue
Vancouver, BC V5Z 4E3, Canada

ARTICLES

The Future of Fibromyalgia:
Some Critical Issues

Frederick Wolfe

SUMMARY. Objectives: To identify issues of importance regarding the validity of the fibromyalgia construct, its pathogenesis, treatment and outcome.

Findings: Major unresolved issues regarding construct, diagnosis, pathogenesis, treatment effect and outcome exist. Confusion between epiphenomena and pathogenetic abnormalities are common. Therapy has not been effective even though statistically significant benefit has been demonstrated.

Conclusions: Future research needs to consider fibromyalgia as a continuum rather than a discrete syndrome or "disease." Pathogenetic studies need to consider psychological factors more prominently. Longitudinal studies of outcome are important. New outcome measures need to be developed.

Frederick Wolfe, MD, is Clinical Professor of Internal Medicine, University of Kansas School of Medicine, Wichita, KS.

Address correspondence to: Frederick Wolfe, MD, Arthritis Research Center, 1035 N. Emporia, STE 230, Wichita, KS 67214.

[Haworth co-indexing entry note]: "The Future of Fibromyalgia: Some Critical Issues." Wolfe, Frederick. Co-published simultaneously in the *Journal of Musculoskeletal Pain* (The Haworth Medical Press, an imprint of The Haworth Press, Inc.) Vol. 3, No. 2, 1995, pp. 3-15; and: *Fibromyalgia, Chronic Fatigue Syndrome, and Repetitive Strain Injury: Current Concepts in Diagnosis, Management, Disability, and Health Economics* (ed: Andrew Chalmers et al.) The Haworth Medical Press, an imprint of The Haworth Press, Inc., 1995, pp. 3-15. Multiple copies of this article/chapter may be purchased from The Haworth Document Delivery Center [1-800-3-HAWORTH; 9:00 a.m. - 5:00 p.m. (EST)].

© 1995 by The Haworth Press, Inc. All rights reserved.

And yet what good were yesterday's devotions?
I affirm and then at midnight the great cat
Leaps quickly from the fireside and is gone.

Montracet-Le-Chardin
Wallace Stevens

YESTERDAY'S DEVOTIONS

The fibromyalgia movement, now spanning two decades, forced to our attention a neglected and large group of patients: those with widespread, almost inexplicable pain, decreased pain threshold, fatigue, sleep disturbance, stiffness, psychological distress, and other symptoms, such as headache, irritable bladder, irritable bowel, subjective swelling, and more. Prior to the fibromyalgia construct, patients with these features were either singled out and diagnosed based on a comprehensible and manageable feature, for example "irritable bowel syndrome," or were diagnosed as having "(osteo)arthritis;" or, even worse, were not considered to have a legitimate complaint, but rather, "psychogenic rheumatism." With the development of criteria, publication in scientific journals, and widespread dissemination of the concept, fibromyalgia achieved a *de facto,* if grudging, recognition: patients with the syndrome abound in the clinic and can be diagnosed easily and with simple criteria. This turn of events had potential for good, for patients' complaints were recognized and physicians began to look into and think about the nature of such complaints. Yet the work of the past decade raises a number of questions.

BUT DOES FIBROMYALGIA EXIST?

In the earlier years of fibromyalgia most studies were descriptive, but increasingly there has been an imperceptible trend to approach the syndrome as if it were a disease. Patient support groups have been formed, manifestos published, and a series of studies performed to unravel the best treatment or to find the cause of fibromyalgia.

Recent epidemiological studies, however, suggest that fibromyalgia symptoms exist in the population as a continuum. Croft reported that as pain increased in the general population from no pain to regional pain to widespread pain, the prevalence of fibromyalgia symptoms [e.g., fatigue, psychological distress, etc.] increased (1). That is, there was a correlation between the topology or extent of pain and the extent and severity of symptoms. Our group approached the problem from another direction (2). We noted associations between pain threshold and fibromyalgia symptoms in the general population: associations that did not depend on a diagnosis of fibromyalgia, but were true across the population at large [Figure 1]. In another study we showed that pain threshold also represents a continuum in the population [Figure 2] (3). In Figure 2, subjects with fibromyalgia represent approximately the 95th percentile of pain threshold. In the clinic, Middleton, studying systemic lupus erythematosus, identified a group with fibromyalgia and then an intermediate group with fewer tender points and fibromyalgia symptoms (4). The thrust of such studies is to suggest that the construct of fibromyalgia may be more properly represented as a continuum than as a discrete syndrome. One important association noted in all of these studies is the correlation between psychological variables and the prevalence of fibromyalgia and fibromyalgia symptoms. Observations about fibromyalgia are analogous to the observations of Pawlikowska et al. concerning the chronic fatigue syndrome [CFS] who wrote " . . . of the continuum of fatiguability . . . " and suggested the CFS " . . . may represent a morbid excess of fatigue rather than a discrete entity, just as high blood pressure and alcohol consumption are morbid ends of normal spectrums" (5).

DOES "PRIMARY" FIBROMYALGIA EXIST [OFTEN]?

"Primary fibromyalgia is said to be fibromyalgia when no other diseases are present that could account for or 'cause' fibromyalgia. The distinction between what is and what is not primary fibromyalgia is difficult. For symptoms and physical findings, patients designated as having primary and secondary or concomitant fibromyalgia do not differ (6); and the ACR 1990 criteria committee abolished the distinction between primary and secondary or concomitant fibromyalgia "at the level of diagnosis" (6). Of interest, population data show an increasing association between age and fibromyalgia [Figure 3]. In the general population the prevalence of fibromyalgia among women is 7.4% [95% confidence limits, 4.8, 10.0] at age 70 and only 0.9% [0.0, 1.7] at age 18-30 (3). The similarity of age vs. prevalence data for fibromyalgia and degenerative disease is striking, suggesting the likelihood of a common relationship. If psychological features were the only or most important feature of fibromyalgia then we would expect a falling off of fibromyalgia prevalence with increasing age since depression, anxiety and family stress tend to decrease in women after age 50 (7). Further support for the idea that "other musculoskeletal

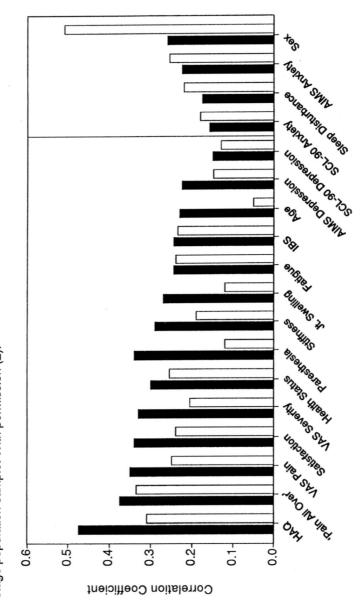

FIGURE 1. Pearson correlation coefficients for the tender point count [solid bars] and dolorimetry scores [clear bars] with fibromyalgia symptoms, psychological status, and demographic characteristics in the general population. Variables to the left of the vertical bar correlate more strongly with the tender point count while variables to the right correlate best with dolorimetry scores. The strongest correlate of digital tenderness is the HAQ score; dolorimetry correlates most strongly with sex. Data are for 391 persons interviewed and examined in the final stage of the two stage population sample. With permission (2).

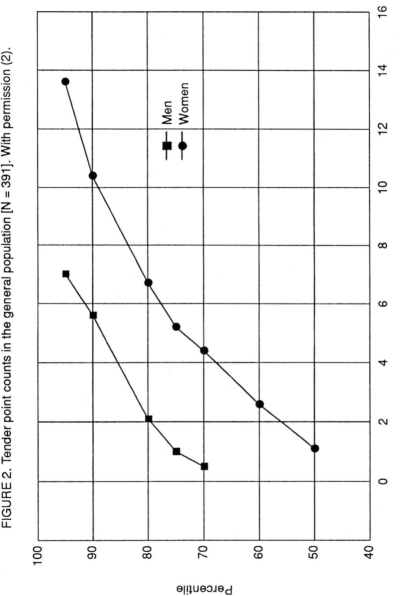

FIGURE 2. Tender point counts in the general population [N = 391]. With permission (2).

7

FIGURE 3. Age and sex specific prevalence of fibromyalgia in the Wichita population for persons aged 18 and above. Circles are women, squares men. Used with permission (3).

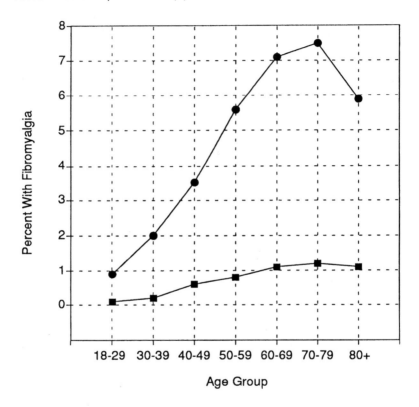

disease" is important comes from the observations that fibromyalgia appears to have an increased prevalence in rheumatoid arthritis and osteoarthritis in the clinic (8,9). Additionally, it has been commonly noted that fibromyalgia occurring in those with other rheumatic complaints seems to exacerbate those *complaints* though not the associated *disease* (10). There are several potential explanations. First, that fibromyalgia is almost always expressed on a substrate of underlying musculoskeletal abnormality, even slight abnormality; and second, that the physical and/or mental stress associated with other significant musculoskeletal disease can exacerbate fibromyalgia. Perhaps, then, true "primary" fibromyalgia is uncommon.

MUST WE USE THE ACR CRITERIA FOR DIAGNOSIS?

The 1990 ACR criteria (6) are useful in their parsimony and simplicity, identifying fibromyalgia by the presence of widespread pain and decreased pain threshold. But it is clear that fibromyalgia is characterized by the presence, in combination, of other features, such as fatigue, sleep disturbance, high levels of pain, irritable bowel syndrome, headache and psychological discomfort, and that in the absence of these features fibromyalgia is unlikely. On a clinical level, diagnosis by a predominance of features has been suggested (11).

The criteria of Table 1 are useful in identifying patients in the clinic who fail to meet the 1990 ACR criteria (6), but who really appear to have the syndrome. To avoid a rigid determinism about what is and what is not fibromyalgia some loosening of the ACR classification criteria are necessary for diagnosis in the clinic. But that same loosening raises questions about the nature of the fibromyalgia construct and the relative importance of tenderness versus "functional" features.

PSYCHOLOGICAL PROBLEMS: YES OR NO?

Fibromyalgia, as it evolved into a medical concept, separated itself from the commonly held view that it represented "psychogenic rheuma-

TABLE 1. Clinical Diagnostic Criteria for Fibromyalgia.

	Non Fibromyalgia Features	Indeterminate Fibromyalgia Features	Characteristic Fibromyalgia Features
Pain	None or limited Pain	Regional to extensive, often with contiguity, but not widespread	Widespread
Tenderness [Tender Points]	0-5	6-10	11 or >
% of Tender points Positive	0-20%	20-55%	> 60%
Symptoms	None or rare	Few to many	Many

Definite fibromyalgia: All of the characteristic fibromyalgia features.
Probable fibromyalgia: Two of the three characteristic fibromyalgia features.
Possible fibromyalgia: One of the three characteristic fibromyalgia features and two of the three indeterminate fibromyalgia features.

tism." While early studies found no psychological abnormality or only a minority of patients with abnormality, with past but not current major depression, most recent studies have shown problems in almost all areas of psychological function. Our group has found depression rates to be 50% greater in fibromyalgia than those with other rheumatic disorders (12), and we have confirmed the finding of increased depression and other problems in a community population survey (3). While recent observations do not "make" fibromyalgia a psychological disorder, they reinforce the importance of psychological factors in the pathogenesis, maintenance, and expression of the syndrome; and they require integration of these findings into other hypotheses of fibromyalgia generation, for psychological factors may be the most important determinant of syndrome expression.

WHAT IS THE MEANING OF LABORATORY ABNORMALITIES IN FIBROMYALGIA?

The last decade has produced a myriad of neurohormonal, neurological and muscle abnormalities. These data are discussed elsewhere in this document. But the central question regarding such findings, besides whether they are reproducible, is whether they are related to how distress and dysfunction are expressed, that is, are secondary or epiphenomena or instead are related in some way to pathogenesis. The former seems more likely since many similar findings are seen in other syndromes. Additionally, such findings beg the issue of their importance because of the likelihood that fibromyalgia is the "morbid" end of a spectrum. There is nothing in the laboratory and/or muscle finding that precludes a major role for psychological factors in pathogenesis of the syndrome.

DOES TREATMENT WORK?

Treatment in fibromyalgia is aimed at several areas: 1. sleep disturbance, 2. musculoskeletal pain, 3. physical and muscular deconditioning, 4. physical measure and 5. psychological and behavioral problems. In a few centers, multidisciplinary specialists use these 5 areas in a continuous treatment program. Treatment of sleep disturbance was undertaken originally because of the EEG sleep abnormality present in fibromyalgia (13,14), and because of the common clinical experience that poor[er] sleep worsens fibromyalgia symptoms. But therapy has been effective only in the short run where some patients show some degree of improvement in a few symptoms or physical finding (15-17). In general, as a rule of thumb, about one-third of patients are improved, but only few substantially. Long-term observations suggest that few patients continue on tricyclic therapy (18), and that long-term controlled trials fail to find benefit (19).

The case is much the same with exercise therapy. Benefit appears to be real, but limited (20). In the real world [as opposed to the clinical trial] few patients obtained the exercise goals set for them. Although in clinical practice one meets patients who are successfully following exercise programs, the numbers are few.

Non-steroidal anti-inflammatory drugs are frequently prescribed, but have not been shown to be effective on fibromyalgia symptoms in controlled trials (17,21). Smythe has suggested the strengthening of the abdominal muscles and the use of a special cervical support pillow improves the symptoms of fibromyalgia (22). These reasonable suggestions have not been subjected to clinical trials.

Recently cognitive-behavioral therapies have been suggested. These psychological approaches to fibromyalgia are now popular, and make sense. Initial reports suggest that such programs might be helpful (23-28), but controlled trials are needed. Cognitive behavioral programs are expensive, not all the same, not all effective, and long-term outcomes are unknown.

Finally, multidisciplinary centers employing all of these approaches have been started. We have suggested elsewhere (29) that "evaluation of such programs is difficult since it is almost impossible to develop adequate controls and because selection processes, compliance, and drop-outs influence results (30), and long-term follow-up is rarely reported (31). In addition, the milieu in which treatment is administered may be more important than the treatment itself" (32).

Early reports have shown variable results. Improvements in psychological measures have been shown. A comprehensive 3 week program reduced depression 47%, trait anxiety 26%, and pain 30% for those completing the program (25). In addition, a number of preliminary positive reports have been published from various centers (27,33-35). But adding physiotherapy to a six-week self-management program was not more effective than self-management alone (36). Why people seem to improve when a "program" is used rather than when the individual components are used is unclear, but it suggests that the continuous nature of the treatment and the psychological support [the "program"] rather than its specific components of the program may be the important factor.

To understand if and when therapy works, and what it costs when it does or doesn't work, longitudinal outcome studies are necessary. It is also necessary to understand what happens to patients with fibromyalgia. Do they get better in the long run? Are they treated for other diagnoses? The limitation of most outcome studies is their short-term nature. Additionally, we may have to measure severity of symptoms better than we do now to understand if patients improve.

WHAT HAPPENS TO PEOPLE WITH FIBROMYALGIA?

Several studies have tracked the outcome of persons with fibromyalgia. Most available data suggest that fibromyalgia is a chronic, rather unchanging disorder that rarely ends in remission (18,37-41). In the most detailed report (40), 4 years after initial examination 97% still had symptoms and 85% fulfilled diagnostic criteria. Fibromyalgia related to trauma also appears to be chronic as well as severe (42). Data like these might lead one to the conclusion that fibromyalgia goes on forever, and that more and more people are afflicted with it. Such a conclusion doesn't quite make sense. Perhaps our follow-up questions are wrong. Because pain is so ubiquitous, do we have a right to expect it to disappear and use that presence or absence as an outcome measure? Perhaps the right measures of outcome are pain severity, function, psychological function and pain behavior. The importance of long-term outcome studies, not only to define outcome but *to define the syndrome,* can not be overestimated.

REFERENCES

1. Croft P, Rigby AS, Boswell R, Schollum J, Silman AJ: The prevalence of widespread pain in the general population. J Rheumatol 20:710-713, 1993.

2. Wolfe F, Ross K, Anderson J, Russell IJ: Aspects of fibromyalgia in the general population: sex, pain threshold, and fibromyalgia symptoms. J Rheumatol 22: 151-156, 1994.

3. Wolfe F, Ross K, Anderson J, Russell IJ, Hebert L: The prevalence and characteristics of fibromyalgia in the general population. Arthritis Rheum 38: 19-28, 1995.

4. Middleton GD, Mcfarlin JE, Lipsky PE: The prevalence and clinical impact of fibromyalgia in systemic lupus erythematosus. Arthritis Rheum 37:1181-1188, 1994.

5. Pawlikowska T, Chalder T, Hirsch SR, Wallace P, Wright DJM, Wessely S: Population based study of fatigue and psychological distress. BMJ 308:763-777, 1994.

6. Wolfe F, Smythe HA, Yunus MB, et al: The American College of Rheumatology 1990 Criteria for the Classification of Fibromyalgia: Report of the Multicenter Criteria Committee. Arthritis Rheum 33:160-172, 1990.

7. Weissman MM, Leaf PJ, Tischler GL, et al: Affective disorders in five United States communities. Psychol Med 18:141-153, 1988.

8. Wolfe F and Cathey MA: Prevalence of primary and secondary fibrositis. J Rheumatol 10:965-968, 1983.

9. Buskila D, Langevitz P, Gladman DD, Urowitz S, Smythe HA: Patients with rheumatoid arthritis are more tender than those with psoriatic arthritis. J Rheumatol 19:1115-1119, 1992.

10. Moldofsky H and Chester WJ: Pain and mood patterns in patients with rheumatoid arthritis. Psychosom Med 32:309-318, 1970.

11. Wolfe F: Fibromyalgia: On diagnosis and certainty. J Musculoske Pain 1(3,4):17-36, 1993.

12. Hawley DJ and Wolfe F: Depression is not more common in rheumatoid arthritis: a 10 year longitudinal study of 6,608 rheumatic disease patients. J Rheumatol 20:2025-2031, 1993.

13. Moldofsky H and Scarisbrick P: Induction of neurasthenic musculoskeletal pain syndrome by selective sleep stage deprivation. Psychosom Med 38:35-44, 1976.

14. Moldofsky H, Scarisbrick P, England R, Smythe HA: Musculoskeletal symptoms and non-REM sleep disturbance in patients with "fibrositis syndrome" and healthy subjects. Psychosom Med 37:341-351, 1975.

15. Bennett RM, Gatter RA, Campbell SM, Andrews RP, Clark SR, Scarola JA: A comparison of cyclobenzaprine and placebo in the management of fibrositis: A double-blind controlled study. Arthritis Rheum 31:1535-1542, 1988.

16. Carette S, McCain GA, Bell DA, Fam AG: Evaluation of amitriptyline in primary fibrositis. A double-blind, placebo-controlled study. Arthritis Rheum 29:655-659, 1986.

17. Goldenberg DL, Felson DT, Dinerman H: A randomized, controlled trial of amitriptyline and naproxen in the treatment of patients with fibromyalgia. Arthritis Rheum 29:1371-1377, 1986.

18. Cathey MA, Wolfe F, Kleinheksel SM, Hawley DJ: Socioeconomic impact of fibrositis. A study of 81 patients with primary fibrositis. Am J Med 81:78-84, 1986.

19. Carette S, Bell MJ, Reynolds WJ, et al: Comparison of Amitriptyline, Cyclobenzaprine, and Placebo in the Treatment of Fibromyalgia–A Randomized, Double-Blind Clinical Trial. Arthritis Rheum 37:32-40, 1994.

20. McCain GA, Bell DA, Mai FM, Halliday PD: A controlled study of the effects of a supervised cardiovascular fitness training program on the manifestations of fibromyalgia. Arthritis Rheum 31:1135-1141, 1988.

21. Yunus MB, Masi AT, Aldag JC: Short term effects of ibuprofen in primary fibromyalgia syndrome: A double blind, placebo controlled trial. J Rheumatol 16:527-532, 1989.

22. Smythe HA: The C6-7 syndrome–Clinical features and treatment response. J Rheumatol 21:1520-1526, 1994.

23. Flor H and Birbaumer N: Comparison of the efficacy of electromyographic biofeedback, cognitive-behavioral therapy, and conservative medical interven-

tions in the treatment of chronic musculoskeletal pain. J Consult Clin Psychol 61:653-658, 1993.

24. Bradley LA: Cognitive-behavioral therapy for primary fibromyalgia. J Rheumatol [Suppl] 19:131-136, 1989.

25. Nielson WR, Walker C, McCain GA: Cognitive Behavioral Treatment of Fibromyalgia Syndrome–Preliminary Findings. J Rheumatol 19:98-103, 1992.

26. Walco GA and Ilowite NT: Cognitive-Behavioral Intervention for Juvenile Primary Fibromyalgia Syndrome. J Rheumatol 19:1617-1619, 1992.

27. Goldenberg DL, Kaplan KH, Nadeau MG, et al: A controlled study of a stress reduction, cognitive–behavioral treatment program in fibromyalgia. J Musculoske Pain 2(2):53-66, 1994.

28. Kaplan KH, Goldenberg DL, Galvinnadeau M: The Impact of a Meditation-Based Stress Reduction Program on Fibromyalgia. Gen Hosp Psychiat 15:284-289, 1993.

29. Wolfe F and Hawley DJ. Fibromyalgia. Edited by WN Kelley, EDJ Harris, S Ruddy, CB Sledge. Textbook of Rheumatology (Supplement). 1993.

30. Turk DC and Rudy TE: Neglected factors in chronic pain treatment outcome studies–Referral patterns, failure to enter treatment, and attrition. Pain 43:7-25, 1990.

31. Turk DC and Rudy TE: Neglected Topics in the Treatment of Chronic Pain Patients-Relapse, Noncompliance, and Adherence Enhancement–Review Article. Pain 44:5-28, 1991.

32. Talo S, Rytokoski U, Puukka P: Patient Classification, a key to evaluate pain treatment: a psychological study in chronic low back pain patients. Spine 17:998-1011, 1992.

33. Burckhardt CS, Clark SR, Campbell SM, O'Reilly CA, Wiens AN, Bennett RM: Multidisciplinary treatment of fibromyalgia. Scand J Rheumatol 21 (Suppl): 51(Abstract).

34. Kogstad O, Hintringer F, Jonsson YM: Patients with fibromyalgia in pain school. J Musculoske Pain 1(3,4):261-265, 1993.

35. de Voogd JN, Knipping AA, De Blecourt ACE, van Rijswijk MH: Treatment of fibromyalgia syndrome with psycho-motor therapy & marital counseling. J Musculoske Pain 1(3,4):273-281, 1993.

36. Burckhardt CS, Mannerkorpi K, Hedenberg L, Bjelle A: A randomized, controlled clinical trial of education and physical training for women with fibromyalgia (FMS). J Rheumatol 21:714-720, 1994.

37. Hawley DJ, Wolfe F, Cathey MA: Pain, functional disability, and psychological status: a 12-month study of severity in fibromyalgia. J Rheumatol 15:1551-1556, 1988.

38. Bengtsson A, Henriksson KG, Jorfeldt L, Kagedal B, Lennmarken C, Lindstrom F: Primary fibromyalgia. A clinical and laboratory study of 55 patients. Scand J Rheumatol 15:340-347, 1986.

39. Felson DT and Goldenberg DL: The natural history of fibromyalgia. Arthritis Rheum 29:1522-1526, 1986.

40. Ledingham J, Doherty S, Doherty M: Primary fibromyalgia syndrome–an outcome study. Brit J Rheumatol 32:139-142, 1993.

41. Henriksson C, Gundmark I, Bengtsson A, Ek AC: Living with Fibromyalgia–Consequences for Everyday Life. Clin J Pain 8:138-144, 1992.

42. Greenfield S, Fitzcharles MA, Esdaile JM: Reactive Fibromyalgia Syndrome. Arthritis Rheum 35:678-681, 1992.

The Chronic Fatigue Syndrome:
An Overview of Important Issues

Irving E. Salit

SUMMARY. There is a sound body of scientific literature on chronic fatigue syndrome [CFS] yet many questions remain. Current evidence does not favor a single infecting agent as the cause. There are probably many factors contributing to the onset and maintenance of CFS. Psychological symptoms are frequent and may be important in the pathogenesis. Minimal investigations are suggested. No single therapy is definitely useful and a multidisciplinary approach is favored. Most patients improve considerably over a period of years.

INTRODUCTION

The chronic fatigue syndrome [CFS] has been investigated from many different aspects and by researchers from varied disciplines. Although this is a refreshing way of approaching any medical problem, in particular CFS, the conclusions derived from these disparate approaches have at times been far-ranging, contradictory and confusing. The scientific and lay literature have resulted in a Tower of Babel syndrome. This can be coun-

Irving E. Salit, MD, is Head of the Division of Infectious Diseases and Director of the Immunodeficiency Clinic, The Toronto Hospital, Toronto, Ontario, Canada.

Address correspondence to: Irving E. Salit, MD, The Toronto Hospital, General Division, 200 Elizabeth Street, Eaton North G-216, Toronto, Ontario, Canada M5G 2C4.

[Haworth co-indexing entry note]: "The Chronic Fatigue Syndrome: An Overview of Important Issues." Salit, Irving E. Co-published simultaneously in the *Journal of Musculoskeletal Pain* (The Haworth Medical Press, an imprint of The Haworth Press, Inc.) Vol. 3, No. 2, 1995, pp. 17-24; and: *Fibromyalgia, Chronic Fatigue Syndrome, and Repetitive Strain Injury: Current Concepts in Diagnosis, Management, Disability, and Health Economics* (ed: Andrew Chalmers et al.) The Haworth Medical Press, an imprint of The Haworth Press, Inc., 1995, pp. 17-24. Multiple copies of this article/chapter may be purchased from The Haworth Document Delivery Center [1-800-3-HAWORTH; 9:00 a.m. - 5:00 p.m. (EST)].

© 1995 by The Haworth Press, Inc. All rights reserved.

terproductive because care providers and patients can select from many different published ideas and approaches; some of these, we believe, may be inhibitory to the fullest possible recovery. In this overview, I will attempt to put some of this information in perspective.

IMPORTANT ISSUES IN CFS

Although good scientific information is accumulating on CFS, there are many uncertainties. CFS usually seems to start rather abruptly, but is this truly the case or is it the patient's perception that it started "out of the blue?" What is the role of preceding psychosocial factors in laying the fertile ground for this sudden onset? The onset of CFS is associated with a variety of triggering factors, but the nature of these factors has not been clearly determined. Even if there is a triggering event for CFS, then one has to explain why the illness often continues for years. The triggering and the maintaining factors may be quite different.

Many diagnostic investigations have been utilized for CFS. These range from very minimal investigations to a variety of sophisticated diagnostic testing which has not been validated for this condition. Patients may travel to CFS centers to have costly testing and other assessments but the relevance of these tests is unknown. Subjects with CFS are managed in many different and contradictory ways [for example, prescribed bedrest vs. exercise], and these different approaches may have profound effects on the maintenance of the illness and its outcome. At this time we do not have good studies on the outcome of CFS which would help to answer some of these questions. Certainly one problem inhibiting those and other studies is the probability that what is included under the rubric of CFS is a number of heterogeneous conditions or at least different subtypes of CFS. It may well be useful to separate these for the purposes of understanding the pathogenesis and for developing optimal approaches to treatment.

I will address below some of these issues in order to highlight the current state of knowledge and to pose questions that we should at least think about and hopefully develop into appropriate research studies.

Precipitating Factors

Major findings. Numerous infective agents have been implicated as the cause of CFS; these include the Epstein-Barr virus, Coxsackie viruses, human herpesvirus-6 [HHV-6], retroviruses, etc. (1). The majority of cases of CFS have no proven association with these or other pathogens (2,3); however, individual cases of CFS have been proven to occur after a variety of infections. I have seen cases in which the precipitating event was documented EBV, Herpes simplex type 2, *Borrelia burgdorferi* [Lyme disease], influenza and *Brucella*. Indeed, brucellosis was a fashionable cause of chronic fatigue about 50 years ago (4). Despite the small number of cases precipitated by a definite infection, almost 75% of people with CFS describe a flu-like illness at the onset of their condition but most do not have a confirmed infection. In the remaining 25% of CFS patients, about half [12%] have another noninfectious precipitating cause such as surgery, allergic reactions or trauma [especially motor vehicle accidents].

Important questions. Since many different infections and also noninfective events seem to be associated with the onset of CFS, it seems most unlikely that any single infection causes the majority of cases. Furthermore, since the infections that have resulted in CFS cause that condition only very rarely then we must either be dealing with an unusual variant of the infection or, much more likely, there is something quite unusual about the patient who gets a common infection yet becomes debilitated. The same can be said for any of the documented precipitating factors. Arguments against a mutant virus with fatigue-producing capabilities include the fact that one would expect more clusters of fatigue, but the opposite occurs: many people within a family have a similar flu-like illness but only one tends to develop the chronic fatigue. Another possibility is that multiple precipitating factors can trigger immunologic or other physiologic changes which would then result in the reactivation of an infecting agent such as a virus; this is a postulated role for HHV-6 (5).

Psychological Factors

Major findings. There are many studies which document high rates of depression during CFS and even preceding its onset (6,7). The severity of the depressive symptoms are frequently intermediate between that seen in major depression and that seen in comparative physical disorders which are associated with fatigue (8). These studies seem to indicate that the depression in CFS is out of proportion to that which can be explained by the disabling fatigue itself. Finally, those presenting with chronic fatigue [of whom only a minority have CFS] also have very high rates of psychiatric disorders (9). Some of the psychiatric disorders frequently associated with chronic fatigue include affective disorders, anxiety and somatization disorders.

Important questions. How are the psychological disorders and CFS related? One possibility is that the fatigue, psychological problems and other symptoms are an intrinsic part of CFS and all are induced and continue because of the same factors. Alternatively, the psychological problems may occur as a result of the physical dysfunction; in this case there is more than one biologic process which is operative. Lastly, one has to consider whether an altered psychological state predisposes to CFS. For example, this could occur by increasing susceptibility to one or more infections or by allowing the symptoms of an infection to persist much longer than they would have otherwise.

Fatigue seems to occur on a continuum in the general population and CFS is one extreme of that condition (10). Given that psychiatric disorders seem to be an explanation for much of the chronic fatigue in the general population, why is the same explanation not valid for CFS?

Test Abnormalities

Major findings. Routine blood tests are generally normal including complete blood count, sedimentation rate and tests of hepatic, renal and thyroid function. However, I commonly note elevation of IgG and/or IgM, an elevation of the CD_4/CD_8 ratio and an elevated 2-5A oligoadenylate synthetase. Other alterations of lymphocyte subsets have been described as well as decreased natural killer cell function (11,12). Immunologic abnormalities are not consistent between studies and are only found in a minority of subjects with CFS. CT brain scans are normal but brain abnormalities have been noted using MRI and SPECT scanning (13,14). Sleep disturbances are very frequent and can be documented in objective sleep studies, but the nature of these abnormalities is quite variable (15,16). Standardized psychological testing has documented a variety of disturbances, including depression and increased stress (6,10). Cognitive dysfunction is a frequent complaint yet objective testing does not consistently demonstrate this abnormality (17). Muscle abnormalities have been noted to be minor or nonexistent (18,19).

Important questions. It would be important to know if there are clear-cut differences in the frequency of the above abnormalities in CFS compared to other conditions such as chronic fatigue, fibromyalgia and psychiatric disorders such as major depression. It is not known if these "abnormalities" are truly abnormalities because of the subjective nature of interpretations or because comparisons have not been made with appropriate controls. Lastly, do observed changes result from an integral part of the pathophysiology of the condition or are they epiphenomena? For example, they may arise as a result of forced disruptions of the patient's usual lifestyle, psychosocial distress, deconditioning, etc.

Management and Outcome

Major findings. Many different therapies have been reported to be beneficial but these have either not been confirmed or have been refuted (20,21,22).

Efamol, magnesium and immunoglobulin injections are not routinely used in clinical practice in part because the experience of the patients and physicians is that they do not work. Patients may attribute improvement, however, to something they have tried because at least some improvement does occur normally over time. We have found that by two years after their initial visit to a tertiary care center, at least half of the patients have improved by 50%; very few are completely well and very few have worsened. It is also rare that any other specific underlying disorder becomes apparent over time. It is important for patients to have this information which should help them to be optimistic about the recovery process.

Important questions. Given the current information on CFS, it seems quite unlikely that a single medication could be completely curative. When physicians and patients have that expectation of a "miracle cure," they can be quite disappointed. Current understanding of CFS indicates a multifactorial causation; with respect to therapy, this implies that a multidisciplinary approach would be quite appropriate. Is this actually the best approach, how should it be done and what are the best ways of comparing treatments and assessing results? Which are the most appropriate measures of the functional state which can be used to determine the results of therapy and to determine disability?

Delineating CFS from Other Conditions

Major findings. CFS overlaps to a great extent with fibromyalgia and major depression (6,7,23). There are several case definitions for CFS and since they do not completely overlap, the diagnosis of CFS is, therefore, variable according to which case definition is applied (24). Furthermore, since there is no diagnostic test for CFS, a definitive diagnosis is not possible.

Important questions. The various case definitions of CFS can reasonably define a syndrome, but can they differentiate CFS from other conditions such as fibromyalgia? This, of course, may not even be a reasonable aim of a case definition because subjects with one of these labels may also have another label. New case definitions for CFS should probably be less restrictive with respect to the requirement for physical findings since they are so infrequent. It should be determined if it is useful to define CFS subgroups based on the nature of the onset [e.g., post-infectious], the presence of psychiatric disorders such as major depression or association with other disorders such as fibromyalgia. Would it not be useful to also include degrees of disability as measured objectively?

Community-Academic Interactions

Major findings. Patients often rely upon newspapers, magazines and community groups for information about CFS. Some of the information in such sources is at variance with the current body of scientific information (25). For example, the lay press may have information on the latest virus which is the apparent cause of CFS, there are claims of instant cures or there is a focus on management strategies which may differ from current suggested approaches by the scientific community.

On the other hand, many physicians do not have an appropriate understanding of the patient's symptoms. Symptoms may be discarded as being "nothing" if there is no physical condition to explain the symptoms. Patients' symptoms are also not taken seriously if it is felt by the physician that they may be psychologically based. CFS patients often come to the physician for a validation of the symptoms but they may be met with skepticism, lack of acceptance and lack of compassion.

Despite ample scientific studies, there is frequently a lack of acceptance of the psychological aspects of the condition by the patients and community groups. Attempts by physicians to discuss psychosocial aspects of the condition can be met with hostility.

Important questions. It is important to determine the reasons for the two solitudes. Why are some physicians so reluctant to accept the patients' symptoms and to work with them to improve their health? Is this due to a lack of understanding of CFS? Is it because of an approach to medicine which separates the mind and body or is it due to a lack of training in managing these types of illnesses? Why are some patients reluctant to examine alternative models of CFS which would include multifactorial causation such as psychosocial factors? Is this due to a stigma attached to psychological disorders?

What are the appropriate clinical approaches which should be used? Should patients use the "rest cure" rather than a graded increase in exercise? Should they stop working in order to avoid as much stress as possible or should they continue on at work, possibly with a reduced load? What are the appropriate approaches to disability assessment and rehabilitation? Physicians and insurance companies on the one hand and the patients and their advocates on the other hand may prefer different approaches.

REFERENCES

1. Salit IE: Sporadic postinfective neuromyasthenia: persistent illness after acute infections. Can Med Ass J. 133:659-663, 1985.

2. Heneine W, Woods TC, Sinha SD, et al: Lack of evidence for infection with known human and animal retroviruses in patients with Chronic Fatigue Syndrome. Clin Infect Dis; 18(Suppl 1): S121-5, 1994.

3. Gow JW, Behan WMH, Simpson K, McGarry F, Keir S, Behan PO: Studies on enterovirus in patients with Chronic Fatigue Syndrome. Clin Infect Dis 18(Suppl 1): S126-9, 1994.

4. Evans AC: Brucellosis in the United States. Am J Public Health 37: 139-151, 1947.

5. Josephs SF, Henry BE, Balachandran N, et al: HHV-6 reactivation in chronic fatigue syndrome. Lancet 337: 1346-1347, 1991.

6. Taerk GS, Toner BA, Salit IE, Garfinkel PE, Ozersky S: Depression in patients with neuromyasthenia (benign myalgic encephalomyelitis). Int J Psychiatry Med 17: 49-56, 1987.

7. Kruesi MJP, Dale JK, Straus SE: Psychiatric diagnoses in patients who have chronic fatigue syndrome. J Clin Psychiatry 50: 53-56, 1989.

8. Wessely S, Powell R: Fatigue syndromes:a comparison of chronic "postviral" fatigue with neuromuscular and affective disorder. J Neurol Neurosurg Psychiatry 52: 940-948, 1989.

9. Manu P, Matthews DA, Lane TJ, et al: Depression among patients with a chief complaint of chronic fatigue. J Affective Disord 17: 165-172, 1989.

10. Pawlikowska T, Chalder T, Hirsch S, Wallace P, Wright D, Wessely S: A population based study of fatigue and psychological distress. Br Med J 308: 763-766, 1994.

11. Landay AL, Jessop C, Lennette ET, Levy JA: Chronic fatigue syndrome: clinical condition associated with immune activation. Lancet 338: 707-712, 1991.

12. Klimas NG, Salvato FR, Morgan R, Fletcher MA: Immunologic abnormalities in chronic fatigue syndrome. J Clin Microbiol 28: 1403-1410, 1990.

13. Ichise M, Salit IE, Abbey SE, et al: Assessment of regional cerebral perfusion by 99Tcm-HMPAO SPECT in chronic fatigue syndrome. Nucl Med Commun 13: 767-772, 1992.

14. Natelson BH, Cohen JM, Brassloff I, Lee H: A controlled study of brain magnetic resonance imaging in patients with the chronic fatigue syndrome. J Neurol Sci 120: 213-217, 1993.

15. Whelton C, Saskin P, Salit H, Moldofsky H: Post-viral fatigue syndrome and sleep. Sleep Res 17: 307, 1988.

16. Krupp LB, Jandorf L, Coyle PK, Mendelson WB: Sleep disturbance in chronic fatigue syndrome. J Psychosom Res 37: 325-331. 1993.

17. Altay HT, Toner BB, Brooker H, Abbey SE, Salit IE, Garfinkel PE: The neuropsychological dimensions of postinfectious neuromyasthenia (chronic fatigue syndrome): a preliminary report. Int. J Psych. in Med 20 (2):141-149, 1990.

18. Lloyd AR, Hales JP, Gandevia SC: Muscle strength, endurance and recovery in the post infection fatigue syndrome. J Neurol Neurosurg Psychiatry 51: 1316-1322, 1988.

19. Stokes MJ, Cooper RG, Edwards RHT: Normal muscle strength and fatiguability in patients with effort syndromes. BMJ 297: 1014-1016, 1988.

20. Straus SE: Intravenous immunoglobulin treatment for the chronic fatigue syndrome. Am J Med 89: 551-552, 1991.

21. Cox IM, Campbell MJ, Dowson D: Red blood cell magnesium and chronic fatigue syndrome. Lancet 337: 757-760, 1991.

22. Behan PO, Behan WMH, Horrobin DF: Effect of high doses of essential fatty acids on the postviral fatigue syndrome. Acta Neurol Scand 82: 209-216, 1990.

23. Goldenberg DL, Simms RW, Geiger A, Komaroff AL: High frequency of fibromyalgia in patients with chronic fatigue seen in a primary care practice. Arthritis Rheum 33: 381-387, 1990.

24. Bates DW, Buchwald D, Lee J, et al: A comparison of case definitions of Chronic Fatigue Syndrome. Clin Infect Dis 18 (Suppl 1): S11-15, 1994.

25. MacLean G, Wessely S: Professional and popular views of chronic fatigue syndrome. Br Med J 308: 776-777, 1994.

Key Issues in Repetitive Strain Injury

Geoffrey O. Littlejohn

SUMMARY. Objective: To examine the nomenclature, clinical features, pathophysiology, management, outcome and prevention of the "RSI" construct, with particular reference to that of fibromyalgia syndrome.

Findings and Conclusion: The condition known as "RSI" is characterized by regional pain and hyperalgesia and other clinical features also seen in generalized fibromyalgia syndrome. The condition is not caused by ongoing tissue damage, is always potentially reversible and like other chronic pain syndromes is influenced by societal and personal factors more than the initial triggering physical and nociceptive factors.

KEYWORDS. RSI, fibromyalgia, work injury

Repetitive strain injury [RSI] is a term devised in the 1980s to describe what was naively thought to be a new medical phenomenon occurring in workplaces throughout the world. RSI referred to the combination of pain, and related symptoms, with disability which was, in the large part, attributed to work practices. Our experience with this problem highlights the

---

Geoffrey O. Littlejohn, MD, MPH, FRACP, FACRM, is Director of Rheumatology and Associate Professor of Medicine, Monash Medical Centre, Monash University, Melbourne, Australia.

Address correspondence to: Dr. Geoffrey Littlejohn, Rheumatology Department, Monash Medical Centre, 246 Clayton Road, Clayton, Victoria, Australia 3168.

[Haworth co-indexing entry note]: "Key Issues in Repetitive Strain Injury." Littlejohn, Geoffrey O. Co-published simultaneously in the *Journal of Musculoskeletal Pain* (The Haworth Medical Press, an imprint of The Haworth Press, Inc.) Vol. 3, No. 2, 1995, pp. 25-33; and: *Fibromyalgia, Chronic Fatigue Syndrome, and Repetitive Strain Injury: Current Concepts in Diagnosis, Management, Disability, and Health Economics* (ed: Andrew Chalmers et al.) The Haworth Medical Press, an imprint of The Haworth Press, Inc., 1995, pp. 25-33. Multiple copies of this article/chapter may be purchased from The Haworth Document Delivery Center [1-800-3-HAWORTH; 9:00 a.m. - 5:00 p.m. (EST)].

© 1995 by The Haworth Press, Inc. All rights reserved.

25

various interacting components of the pain system–those which range from nociceptor stimulation through to societal and cultural influences on pain complaint. In certain countries, RSI presented as a significant epidemic which has largely resolved. However, increasing rates of RSI are now reported in other countries. The cost to the individual, their family, the community and the country in which they live is extraordinarily high. The difficulties of management of the individual with the RSI problem must be contrasted with the observations made when one overviews the situation. This review focuses on several key issues which relate to the RSI problem. The bottom line is that the problem is manageable even before explanatory pathophysiological factors are fully understood.

THE PROBLEM–WHAT IS IT?

There is confusion as to what the term RSI actually describes. This has led to altered beliefs of the public and health care professionals alike as to the nature of symptoms which occur with activity of the musculoskeletal system. The general notion is that the "RSI" symptoms reflect ongoing activity-related injurious nociceptor stimulation of one of the components of a muscle-tendon unit. However, this is far from the case.

The various components of the muscle-tendon unit comprise muscle, muscle-tendon junction and paratenon region, tendon, tendon sheath, and the enthesial regions which bind the tendon, ligament or joint capsule to bone. All of these components may be subject to activity-related strain or sprain. With persistent use degenerative change might occur. As a consequence of such tissue damage, inflammatory and repair mechanisms may be activated leading to a defined disorder of one of the components of the muscle-tendon unit. As the prime movers of the musculoskeletal system, such regions are under a lot of physical stress. They are also highly innervated with nociceptor fibers. Excessive activity, be it on an everyday or an episodic basis, will result in clinical features which denote a wide range of well-recognized disorders of the muscle-tendon unit. These include muscle strain, tenosynovitis or enthesitis. Nerve root entrapment syndromes may occur.

The cause of these problems is well-defined and usually obvious. The outcome relates to the background state of the tissues and the extent of the activity-related tissue damage. Each tissue has a different threshold for injury. The treatment and outcome programs are fairly predictable and relate to our understanding of tissue damage. Preventive work programs require knowledge of the response of the muscle-tendon unit to various ergonomic demands.

It was hoped that the term RSI would usefully encompass all of the above types of conditions. However, as evidenced by the Australian epidemic of RSI, the nature of the continuing complaint of pain and disability was actually different to that which defined one of the well-known and named problems affecting the muscle-tendon unit (1). The RSI problem did not consistently associate with ergonomic observations, nor respond to standard treatments which would resolve an inflammatory or degenerative condition of the muscle-tendon unit. The pain persisted and spread from the original region of complaint to involve the entire limb, including neck and chest wall and often the opposite limb. The upper limb was the main area of complaint. The limb became hyperalgesic, particularly so in the fibromyalgia tender point regions. Muscular co-contraction, allodynia, decreased muscular compliance, subcutaneous swelling, peripheral dysesthesia [without anatomical signs] and vasomotor changes also occurred (1,2).

The majority of patients with the "RSI problem" have a chronic pain syndrome which, although it may be triggered by a simple injury to the muscle-tendon unit, is not due to persisting tissue damage or injury. Extensive investigation seeking out tissue damage and injury will only show age-related or incidental changes which do not explain the diffuse symptoms.

NOMENCLATURE

The use of the term RSI is inappropriate and should be avoided. In this review the term is used only as a starting point. RSI is typical of a number of names applied to chronic pain syndromes which imply causation. Where the pain is localized a variety of naive labels are used. These include railway spine, whiplash syndrome, Mediterranean back and other pejorative and confusing terms. RSI was coined during the early stages of the Australian epidemic of regional arm pain. Other equally unacceptable terms for the same condition include occupational overuse syndrome, cumulative trauma disorder or occupational cervico-brachial disorder.

In the mid-1980s, during the Australian "RSI" epidemic the Royal Australasian College of Physicians lobbied to change the name to a descriptive title, that of regional pain syndrome. Such approaches were helpful in changing the communities' belief in regard to the nature of the problem. This author favors a mechanistic descriptive term, that of localized fibromyalgia, because of the identical clinical features and the fact that generalized fibromyalgia syndrome often follows. It is important to separate this localized pain syndrome from myofascial pain syndromes with their peripheral nociceptive stimulus. As our knowledge increases better terms will be used. [Table 1].

CLINICAL FEATURES

What then are the clinical features of localized fibromyalgia? Basically they are the same as generalized fibromyalgia except that the pain and clinical features are regionalized. The core clinical features are those of regionalized pain and hyperalgesia, fatigue, poor sleep and emotional distress. These are the same five core features seen in generalized fibromyalgia. In localized fibromyalgia there will be regionalized proximal muscle co-contraction, muscular stiffness, non-anatomical dysesthesia, vasomotor changes and dermatographia. These clinical features vary in intensity among subjects. The upper limb pain and hyperalgesia are inevitably associated with disability. No validated classification or diagnostic criteria exist but operational criteria appear useful in clinical practice [Table 2].

PATHOPHYSIOLOGY

The pathophysiology of this process has still to be clarified. The following synopsis reviews processes which appear to be relevant. Presumably,

TABLE 1. Nomenclature for "RSI"

1.	**Tissue Damage to Component of Muscle-Tendon Unit**	
	Site	– e.g. hand
	Specific component involved	– flexor tendon sheath
	Type of pathophysiological process	– inflammation
		= "flexor tenosynovitis of hand"
2.	**No Ongoing Tissue Damage–PAIN SYNDROME**	
[i]	**Non-Acceptable Nomenclature**	
	Repetitive Strain Injury, Syndrome	[RSI]
	Occupational Overuse Syndrome	[OOS]
	Cumulative Trauma Disorder	[CTD]
	Occupational Cervicobrachial Disorder	[OCD]
[ii]	**Acceptable Nomenclature**	
	Descriptive	Regional Pain Syndrome
	Mechanistic	Localized Fibromyalgia Syndrome
	Pathophysiological	Sensitization with Secondary Hyperalgesia

TABLE 2. Operational Criteria for Localized Fibromyalgia

1.	Regional pain
2.	Regional hyperalgesia [including regional tender points, 6 maximum ACR for upper limb, others often present]
3.	Sleep disorder
4.	Fatigue
5.	Emotional distress
6.	No other identified cause of axial/peripheral nonciception to explain diffuse symptoms/signs

in the first instance, there is an activity-related stimulus to a nociceptor in one of the susceptible muscle-tendon unit regions. This may be proximal, for instance, in and around the region of the neck, or distal, for instance, in the tendon sheaths of the hand. It may also be superficial, where the pain would be perceived locally, or the stimulus may be deep, where reflex "referred" pain mechanisms would be initiated. With increased activity the nociceptor threshold will be lower in one of the above regions and an electrical stimulus will be initiated. Where repetitive peripheral nociceptive stimuli impinge on the dorsal horn, the mechanism of "windup" might be involved (3).

Of more importance than these peripheral mechanisms are central mechanisms, although both are intimately related. Modulation of the function of dorsal horn pain transmission neurons may cause sensitization, a process whereby previously subthreshold stimuli now produce action potentials. Through descending pathways from higher centers, a variety of "psychological" factors, such as sleep disturbance, personality, emotion, mood and beliefs may play a role in changing dorsal horn transmission cell function in any one individual.

Dorsal horn neurons include not only specific nociceptive neurons but also wide dynamic range neurons which receive input from nociceptor fibers and also mechanoreceptor fibers. Normal impulses coming via the mechanoreceptor system will feed afferent information which was previously subthreshold into this sensitized pain transmission neuron. Through this change in function, routine movements or postures, particularly those involving regions which are highly innervated with mechanoreceptors, become painful. Mechanoreceptor innervation is particularly high around facet joints and related structures. Because of the unique postural characteristics of the low cervical spine and the adjacent locality of the upper limb, there is more afferent information coming from these mechanoreceptors than from others in adjacent areas. With amplification of the pain system, through sensitization of the pain transmission neurons, this information is translated into pain complaint and clinical signs which preferentially relate to the low cervical spine area of reference. In addition, it is common to find altered range of motion or localized tenderness in the low cervical spines of normal asymptomatic subjects. Such situations have been termed vertebral dysfunctions. These sites also provide increased mechanoreceptor input and may associate with certain work, recreational or sleep postures. Vertebral dysfunctions are associated with both localized and generalized fibromyalgia syndrome (4).

When these deeper paravertebral structures provide increased afferent "input" to the dorsal horn, then various reflex phenomena, involved in the process of the "referred pain," come into play. "Referred pain" consists of symptoms such as deep aching, skin tenderness, regionalized hyperalgesia [more prominent in the tender points, as also occurs in pain free persons (5)], dysesthesia, swelling and allodynia, among others. The sensitized pain transmission neurons result in expansion of receptive fields leading to spread of the pain complaint and regional hyperalgesia. The resulting symptoms comprise spontaneous pain, spread of pain and reflex muscle tightness, as well as the clinical findings of hyperalgesia, among others.

Sensitization of the peripheral nociceptor accompanies sensitization of the dorsal horn pain transmission neurons. Activity within the A-delta and C afferent fibers, which largely subserve the function of nociception, is increased in localized fibromyalgia syndrome. Neurotransmitters, including substance P, are released on stimulation of C fibers and result in neurogenic inflammation (6). This process may cause some of the clinical features of localized fibromyalgia, such as dermatographia, allodynia, and swelling and may contribute to complaints of pain. Neuropeptides also sensitize peripheral nociceptor fibers which will also involve deeply placed structures such as facet joints and related structures, which in turn leads to "referred pain."

Comparison with phantom limb phenomena and consideration of the neuromatrix theory (7) may be relevant to this regionalized pain complaint. The sympathetic nervous system is also activated in many patients with regionalized pain syndromes, just as it is in generalized fibromyalgia syndrome (8). This may further modulate the peripheral pain system through sensitization of the afferent nerve ending, but will also act centrally. It is interesting to speculate on the often rapid development of regionalized pain syndromes, perhaps suggesting that secretion of centrally-placed neuromodulators, such as corticotrophin releasing hormone, have a possible role.

While the exact pathophysiology of regionalized pain syndromes has not been deduced, the essential and important point is that there is no evidence to suggest a peripheral tissue damage cause for the complaint and much evidence to suggest that sensitization of the pain system is intrinsic to the persistence of pain and other clinical features. This has major implications in regard to preventive and management programs.

MANAGEMENT

Management of regional pain complaints such as localized fibromyalgia may be misdirected. If the situation is managed as an injury, numerous investigations will follow seeking to document the extent or nature of the perceived injury. This may include excessive use of imaging, nerve conduction studies, thermography or blood tests. Usually the patient is supported by a third party provider in such situations, and is non-discriminatory in regard to which tests might be recommended. The persisting complaint of pain with its pressing need to be relieved and understood often leads to a very permissive investigation profile, financially beneficial to some but detrimental to the patient.

In this setting the injury model is often inappropriately used. This leads to the notion that the patient has a serious and difficult to diagnose injurious condition which evades the best of medical science. The patient is advised to rest until the problem "gets better." Numerous interventions occur which often persist for weeks or months, even years, despite lack of useful benefit. Off-work certification results and medico-legal issues enter. The patient is in pain, disabled and confused. Financial security becomes an issue and dispute as to the "reality" of the syndrome enters the picture.

In contrast, if the problem is seen and managed as a pain syndrome then the outcome can be expected to be good. The patient is not advised to rest, early return to work is suggested, excessive physical treatments are avoided and only simple analgesic and sleep modification medication may be prescribed. A satisfactory education program involving the patient, family, workplace and society in general is necessary. Various psychological modulating therapies may be necessary.

OUTCOME

The outcome of this syndrome is highlighted by reflection on the Australian experience through the 1980s. There has been a return to the low endemic rates of the early 80s after a dramatic peak through the mid-1980s of significant workplace-associated upper arm pain and disability (1). Despite intensive litigation, compensation and publicity at the time, most persons are now back at work, many at their previous job doing the same activity and using the same equipment (9). In Australia persons who have had "RSI" now seldom talk of it. Patients are not continuing to see doctors for persistent regionalized pain complaints unless there is an outstanding medico-legal or psychosocial issue which is unresolved. This is not to say that all symptoms disappear, but it does say that the severity of the complaint diminishes significantly and most persons can return to a normal or near normal lifestyle.

These facts are extremely important when assessing an individual with the problem. The intense medico-legal and psychosocial pressures promote further stress which, when removed, allow appropriate management strategies to be remarkably effective. Such strategies demand co-operation and insight from the patient, as they are the key leaders of the treatment team.

PREVENTION

Social inputs influence the reporting and are part of the pathogenesis of regionalized pain complaints such as "RSI." The Australian epidemic diminished through publicity about the nature of the problem, legal determinations which rejected the notion of persistence of injury, and increased social awareness as to the nature of the problem. It became unfashionable to have RSI. In some situations it was falsely equated to "malingering," with resultant stigmatization. During the epidemic, persons were encouraged to report minor symptoms through intensive union-promoted publicity. Today, the publicity from Australian workers compensation organizations encourages people to "stay at work–work is good for you even if you are injured." Minor complaints are treated seriously and with common sense medical ergonomic principles. They are no longer the first step in a chain of events that allows for pain amplification. Judicious use of legislation and other socio-cultural factors play an important role in prevention and management of chronic pain syndromes.

Knowledge of fibromyalgia and chronic pain syndromes is a necessary postgraduate skill required for all rehabilitation and primary care health personnel. This knowledge should be used together with identification of injury-associated ergonomic triggers in the workplace, early accurate diagnosis and management of specific, named muscle-tendon unit injury problems, recognition of pain modulation, education of the community, appropriate recognition and care of the person who has developed localized fibromyalgia and review of permissive legislation. The social iatrogenicity induced by medico-legal aspects of this problem is high.

Thus, in summary, "RSI" is seen as a complex pathophysiological pain problem whose clinical features may be approached using the paradigm of localized fibromyalgia syndrome. Ergonomic triggering factors together with personal and societal factors induce physiological changes which cause the person's pain complaint and disability. Despite all the difficulties which such situations bring "RSI" is manageable even with our current limited knowledge of chronic pain mechanisms.

REFERENCES

1. Littlejohn GO: Repetitive strain syndrome, Rheumatology. Edited by JH Klippel and P Dieppe, Mosby-Year Book Europe Ltd, London, 1994, section 5, pp. 17.1-17.5.

2. Littlejohn GO: Repetitive strain syndrome: an Australian experience. J Rheumatol 13: 1004-1006, 1986.

3. Mendell LM: Physiological properties of unmyelinated fiber projections to the spinal cord. Exp Neurol 16: 316-332, 1966.

4. Granges G, Littlejohn GO: Postural and mechanical factors in localized and generalized fibromyalgia/fibrositis syndrome. Progress in Myofascial Pain and Fibromyalgia. Edited by H Vaeroy and H Merskey, Elsevier Science Publishers, Amsterdam, 1993, pp. 329-348.

5. Granges G, Littlejohn GO: Pressure pain threshold in pain free subjects, in patients with chronic regional pain syndromes and in fibromyalgia syndrome. Arthritis Rheum 36: 642-646, 1993.

6. Chahl LA, Szolcsanyi J, Lembeck F: Antidromic vasodilatation and neurogenic inflammation. Budapet Akademiai Kiado, 1984.

7. Coderre TJ, Katz J, Vaccarion AL, Melzack R: Contribution of central neuroplasticity to pathological pain: review of clinical and experimental evidence. Pain 52: 259-285, 1993.

8. Vaeroy H, Qiao ZG, Morkid L, Forre O: Altered sympathetic nervous system response in patients with fibromyalgia [fibrositis syndrome]. J Rheumatol 16: 1460-1465, 1989.

9. Travers R: Soft-tissue rheumatism in industry. Rev Espan de Reum 20 (suppl 1): 251-252, 1993.

Aspects of the Pathogenesis of Chronic Muscular Pain

Karl G. Henriksson

SUMMARY. Objectives: To give an overview of investigations that have increased our understanding of the pathogenesis of chronic generalized muscular pain and hyperalgesia [tender points] in the fibromyalgia syndrome [FS] and in chronic fatigue syndrome [CFS].

Results and Conclusions: The results of current research support the following hypothesis that includes both peripheral [muscular] and central factors. The changes in the central nociceptive system that leads to central sensitization of nociceptive neurons are probably the specific features of muscular pain in FS and CFS. The muscular changes indicating a localized disturbance of microcirculation, which can excite and sensitize nociceptors in the muscle, represent promoting or triggering factors and are not specific for fibromyalgia.

KEYWORDS. Fibromyalgia, muscle pain, nociception, hyperalgesia

CLINICAL ASPECTS

Muscular pain caused by mechanical trauma, by overstretching [e.g., in postexertional pain] or by a metabolic disturbance [e.g., phosphorylase,

---

Karl G. Henriksson, MD, PhD, is Associate Professor in Neurology, The University Hospital, Linköping, Sweden.

[Haworth co-indexing entry note]: "Aspects of the Pathogenesis of Chronic Muscular Pain." Henriksson, Karl G. Co-published simultaneously in the *Journal of Musculoskeletal Pain* (The Haworth Medical Press, an imprint of The Haworth Press, Inc.) Vol. 3, No. 2, 1995, pp. 35-41; and: *Fibromyalgia, Chronic Fatigue Syndrome, and Repetitive Strain Injury: Current Concepts in Diagnosis, Management, Disability, and Health Economics* (ed: Andrew Chalmers et al.) The Haworth Medical Press, an imprint of The Haworth Press, Inc., 1995, pp. 35-41. Multiple copies of this article/chapter may be purchased from The Haworth Document Delivery Center [1-800-3-HAWORTH; 9:00 a.m. - 5:00 p.m. (EST)].

© 1995 by The Haworth Press, Inc. All rights reserved.

carnitine palmiotyltransferase and myoadenylate deaminase deficiency] is a pain on exertion. Pain is absent at muscular rest. Inflammation in the muscle is sometimes but not always painful (1).

If nerve fascicles to a muscle are stimulated, the pain elicited has an aching, cramp-like character and a more diffuse delineation than pain in the skin (2,3,4).

Koltzenburg, LaMotte, and Torebjörk and their coworkers (5,6,7) have studied hyperalgesia in awake human subjects with microneurography. A localized tissue damage in the skin was caused by the injection of capsaicin or the application of mustard oil. Primary hyperalgesia, i.e., hyperalgesia within the area of tissue damage developed as did secondary hyperalgesia, i.e., hyperalgesia in the area surrounding the damaged area. The primary hyperalgesia was due to impulses in nociceptive C fibers. The secondary hyperalgesia was due to changes in the central nociceptive system. It was shown that impulses in afferent nerves from the periphery were a prerequisite not only for the peripheral, but also for central sensitization of nociceptive nerves. We do not know if the mechanisms for hyperalgesia in muscle [tender points] are the same as in the skin and we do not know whether mechanisms for chronic hyperalgesia are the same as in acute hyperalgesia, but we do know that tender points and pain in patients with FS disappear if the impulse traffic in afferent nerves is blocked, e.g., during epidural blockade (8).

In FS and in those patients with CFS who have generalized pain and hyperalgesia, there is muscular pain at muscular rest. The pain is often continuous. In 78% of patients with FS the pain was present during 95% of time awake (9). It is often diminished during moderate exercise, but gets worse after exercise. The pain after exercise can last several hours, and is not segmental or regional but generalized to all four body quadrants. It is most often described as aching but it is common that the pain also has other characteristics, such as burning. The hyperalgesia [allodynia] to moderate pressure at many locations is chronic and the tender points are found in both the upper and lower halves of the body.

All these clinical features in FS point to a disturbance in the nociceptive system in the CNS, not to muscle. It cannot be excluded, however, that muscular changes are important for development and for maintaining the central changes. This will be discussed below.

THE CENTRAL NOCICEPTIVE SYSTEM

Impulses in primary afferent nociceptive nerves can either be amplified or inhibited at different levels in the CNS. It has been shown in animal experiments that impulses in primary nociceptive nerves from muscle are more strongly inhibited than, for example, impulses in nociceptor nerves from the skin. Damage to descending inhibitory pathways results in increased resting activity and an amplification of the response to noxious stimulation. There is also an increased convergence of impulses from different receptors and an increase of the number of receptive fields [see review article by Mense for references (10,11)].

Serotonin is an important transmitter substance in descending inhibitory pathways. It is of interest in this context that aberrations in serotonin metabolism have been found in patients with FS (12,13,14). In a German investigation, 74% of patients with FS had antibodies against serotonin and gangliosides (15). The authors discussed the possibility that these antibodies are against serotonin receptors. In patients where excessive fatigue dominates over pain and where the pain is generalized from the onset, neuroendocrinological abberations may be of more importance for the pathogenesis than in patients where the pain is localized at onset and where there is a slow transition to generalized pain.

REFERRAL OF MUSCULAR PAIN

The prevailing theory is that of convergence-projection which means that nerve impulses in afferent nerve fibers from the skin, from deep tissues and internal organs converge on the same dorsal horn nerve cell. Mense has recently reviewed his own and others' experimental findings and emphasized two other aspects (11). Firstly, there is support for the possibility that noxious stimuli to the muscle can open new convergent connections. Secondly, and relevant for the understanding of the generalization of pain in FS, central sensitization may spread to several segments due to diffusion of neuropeptides like substance P within the dorsal horn (11).

The question is whether the changes in the central nociceptive system are secondary to longstanding bombardment of the CNS by impulses in primary nociceptive nerves from muscles, tendon, ligaments etc., or if they are a part of an immunological or neuroendocrinological disturbance. Bennett et al., in animal experiments, have found that impulses in nociceptive nerves caused by partial nerve lesions can damage neurons in the dorsal horn (16). It should not be excluded that the pathogenesis of the central sensitization could be different in different patients.

The studies that support the presence of a neurogenic inflammation in FS indicate that there is an activation of primary pain neurons (17). Neurogenic inflammation is caused by neuropeptides that cause, e.g., degranulation of mast cells. One important neuropeptide involved in neurogenic inflammation is substance P. This is produced in dorsal root ganglia, from which it is transported antidromically to the nerve endings and to a lesser extent centrally to the dorsal horn and CSF. An increased amount of connective tissue mast cells in the skin and increased amount of substance P in the CSF (18,19) are findings in patients with FS. These findings support the notion that there is activity in primary nociceptive neurons in FS.

So far, changes that could cause excitation and sensitization of nociceptors have been found only in the muscle. The tendons and ligaments have not been investigated. The muscular changes that will be described below should be regarded as significant for pain and hyperalgesia, as they can be related to factors that excite and/or sensitize nociceptors in the muscle.

THE MUSCULAR CHANGES

The morphological, biochemical and physiological changes described in some muscles like the trapezius muscle in patients with FS or chronic trapezius myalgia are fairly discrete. They are not detected in magnetic resonance spectroscopy studies, a method in this context with too low a power of resolution (20). A disturbance of microcirculation with focal hypoxia or accumulation of algogenic substances is the most likely cause of excitation and sensitization of intramuscular nociceptors. There are findings that support a disturbed microcirculation in some muscles both in FS and in chronic localized myalgia (21-26). It should be emphasized that some of these findings can even be seen in persons with no pain. The difference between persons with pain and persons without pain may be more quantitative than qualitative.

What then is the cause of chronic disturbance of microcirculation in some muscles? Elerts' studies show that FS patients had insufficient relaxation of muscles between muscle contractions (27). The degree of muscle tension in the rest period between contractions was high enough to affect intramuscular microcirculation. A faulty central motor control ["bad motor habits"] could be one explanation.

The muscular changes could be described as microlesions. Bennett (28) discusses also the possibility that microtrauma secondary to inactivity could be a factor that could give pain. His and his coworkers' finding that patients with FS have lower somatomedin C values than controls indicates a decreased release of growth hormone and is of interest in this context as this could mean a deficient repair of microlesions or microtrauma that occurs in all of us as a result of ordinary muscle use and overuse (29).

MUSCLE TENSION

A feeling of increased muscle tension or stiffness is often reported by patients with FS. Muscle tension is not equivalent to pain. The question is whether nerve impulses from the muscle that normally are perceived as tension will be perceived as pain if there is sensitization of central nociceptive neurons (30).

REFERENCES

1. Henriksson KG, Sandstedt P: Polymyositis–treatment and prognosis. A study of 107 patients. Acta Neurol Scand 65: 280-300, 1982.

2. Torebjörk HE, Ochoa JL, Schady W: Referred Pain from Intraneural Stimulation of Muscle Fascicles in the Median Nerve. Pain 18: 145-156, 1984.

3. Simone DA, Caputi G, Marchettini P, Ochoa J: Muscle nociceptors identified in humans; intraneural recordings, microstimulation and pain. Soc Neurosci Abst 17: 546, 1991.

4. Marchettini P, Ochoa J: The Clinical Implications of Referred Muscle Pain Sensation. APS Journal 3(1): 10-12, 1994.

5. Koltzenburg M, Lundberg LER, Torebjörk HE: Dynamic and static components of mechanical hyperalgesia in human hairy skin. Pain 51: 207-219, 1992.

6. Torebjörk HE, Lundberg LER, Lamotte RH: Central changes in processing of mechanoreceptive input in capsaicin-induced secondary hyperalgesia in humans. J Physiol 448: 765-780, 1992.

7. La Motte RH, Lundberg LE, Torebjörk HE: Pain, hyperalgesia and activity in nociceptive C units in humans after intradermal injection of capsaicin. J Physiol 448: 749-764, 1992.

8. Bengtsson M, Bengtsson A, Jorfeldt L: Diagnostic epidural opioid blockade in primary fibromyalgia at rest and during exercise. Pain 39: 171-180, 1989.

9. Henriksson Chris, Gundmark I, Bengtsson A, Ek A-Ch: Living with fibromyalgia. Consequences for everyday life. Clinc J Pain 8: 138-144, 1992.

10. Mense S: Nociception from skeletal muscle in relation to clinical muscle pain. Review Article. Pain 54: 241-289, 1993.

11. Mense S: Referral of Muscle Pain. New Aspects. APS Journal 3(1): 1-9, 1994.

12. Russell IJ, Værøy H, Javors M, Nyberg F: Cerebrospinal fluid biogenic amine metabolites in fibromyalgia/fibrositis syndrome and rheumatoid arthritis. Arthritis and Rheumatism 35: 550-556, 1992 b.

13. Russell IJ, Bowden CL, Michalek J: Platelet ^{3}H-imipramine uptake receptor density and serum serotonin levels in patients with fibromyalgia/fibrositis syndrome. J Rheumatol 19: 104-109, 1992.

14. Yunus MB, Dailey JW, Masi AT, Jobe PC: Plasma tryptophan and other amino acids in primary fibromyalgia: a controlled study. J Rheumatol 19:9: 90-94, 1992.

15. Klein R, Bänsch M, Berg PA: Clinical relevance of antibodies against serotonin and gangliosides in patients with primary fibromyalgia syndrome. Psychoneuroendocrinology 17:6: 593-598, 1992.

16. Bennett GJ, Kajander KC, Sahara Y, Iadarola MJ, Sugimoto T: Neurochemical and anatomical changes in the dorsal horn of rats with an experimental painful peripheral neuropathy. In F Cervero, GJ Bennett, P Headley (eds.) Processing of Sensory Information in the Superficial Dorsal Horn of Spinal Cord. pp. 463-471. vol 176, Plenum, New York, 1989.

17. Littlejohn GO, Weinstein C, Helme RD: Increased Neurogenic Inflammation in Fibrositis Syndrome. J Rheumatol 14:5: 1022-1025, 1987.

18. Eneström S, Bengtsson A, Lindström F, Johan K: Attachment of IgG to dermal extracellular matrix in patients with fibromyalgia. Clin and Experimental Rheumatol 8: 127-135, 1990.

19. Værøy H, Helle R, Øystein F, Kåss E, Terenius L: Elevated CSF levels of substance P and high incidence of Raynaud phenomenon in patients with fibromyalgia; new features for diagnosis. Pain 32: 21-26, 1988.

20. Simms RW, Roy S, Hrovat M, Anderson JJ, Skrinar G, et al: Fibromyalgia syndrome (FMSS) is not associated with abnormalities in muscle energy metabolism. Scand J Rheumatol Suppl 94: 19, 1992.

21. Lund N, Bengtsson A, Thorborg P: Muscle Tissue Oxygen Pressure in Primary Fibromyalgia. Scand J Rheum 15: 165-173, 1986.

22. Larsson SE, Bodegård L, Henriksson KG, Öberg PÅ: Chronic trapezius myalgia. Morphology and blood flow studied in 17 patients. Acta Orthop Scand 61(5): 394-398, 1990.

23. Larsson S-E, Ålund M, Hongming C, Öberg PÅ: Chronic Pain after soft-tissue injury of the cervical spine. Trapezius muscle blood flow and electromyography at static loads and fatigue. Pain (accepted for publication), 1994.

24. Henriksson KG, Bengtsson A, Lindman R, Thornell LE: Morphological changes in muscle in fibromyalgia and chronic shoulder myalgia. In Merskey H, Væroy H (eds.) Progress in fibromyalgia and Myofascial Pain. Elsevier Science Publishers, 1993.

25. Lindman R, Hagberg M, Bengtsson A, Henriksson KG, Thornell LE: Changes in Trapezius Muscel Structure in Fibromyalgia and Chronic Trapezius Myalgia. J Musculoskeletal Pain 1(3/4): 171-176, 1993.

26. Bengtsson A, Bengtsson M: Regional sympathetic blockade in primary fibromyalgia. Pain 33: 161-167, 1988.

27. Elert JE, Rantapää-Dahlqvist SB, Henriksson-Larsén K, Gerdle BUC: Increased EMG activity during short pauses in patients with primary fibromyalgia. Scand J Rheuamtol 18: 321-323, 1989.

28. Bennett RM: The origin of myopain: An intergrated hypothesis of focal muscle changes and sleep disturbance in patients with the fibromyalgia syndrome. J Musculoskeletal Pain 1(3/4): 95-112, 1993.

29. Bennett RM, Clark SR, Campbell SM, Burckhardt CS: Low levels of somatomedin C in patients with the fibromyalgia syndrome. A possible link be-

tween sleep and muscle pain. Arthritis and Rheumatism 35:10: 1113-1116, 1992.

30. Johansson H, Sojka P: Pathophysiological mechanisms involved in genesis and spread of muscular tension in occupational muscle pain and in chronic musculoskeletal pain syndromes. A hypothesis. Med Hypotheses 35: 196-203, 1991.

Fibromyalgia–
A Historical Perspective

Anthony S. Russell

While I think there have been a number of gains from the codifying and delineation of fibromyalgia [FS], there are also some questions to be asked. The diagnosis, at least as it appears in clinic patients, seems robust. Follow up several years later shows patients to be symptomatic but with no change in the nature of their underlying disorder. On the other hand, those patients detected by questionnaires in the general population have milder and much more fluctuating symptoms. The main question I think is: is FS a disease, albeit with several etiologies and perhaps pathogenetic pathways, or is FS a behavior disorder supported, and often stimulated, by societal and medical fashions? As has been pointed out before (1), the disorder does not have much "face validity." Patients with chronic pain put themselves, by self-reported questionnaire (2), in a category of disability second only to amyotrophic lateral sclerosis, far worse than rheumatoid arthritis, colitis, etc. This degree of disability clearly seems at variance with the physical signs, although not always with the patient's behavior. One great advantage of defining and codifying this problem is that at the level of the individual patient it has called a halt to the never-ending searches for obscure organic disease–"Furor Medicus"–thus it allows a positive diagnosis to be made without the time and expense of a diagnosis of exclusion. I do not accept the views of 2 representatives from the Copenhagen conference who are quoted as saying that many patients will

Anthony S. Russell, FRCP[C], is Professor of Medicine, University of Alberta, 562 Heritage Medical Research Centre, Edmonton, Alberta, Canada T6G 2S2.

[Haworth co-indexing entry note]: "Fibromyalgia–A Historical Perspective." Russell, Anthony S. Co-published simultaneously in the *Journal of Musculoskeletal Pain* (The Haworth Medical Press, an imprint of The Haworth Press, Inc.) Vol. 3, No. 2, 1995, pp. 43-48; and: *Fibromyalgia, Chronic Fatigue Syndrome, and Repetitive Strain Injury: Current Concepts in Diagnosis, Management, Disability, and Health Economics* (ed: Andrew Chalmers et al.) The Haworth Medical Press, an imprint of The Haworth Press, Inc., 1995, pp. 43-48. Multiple copies of this article/chapter may be purchased from The Haworth Document Delivery Center [1-800-3-HAWORTH; 9:00 a.m. - 5:00 p.m. (EST)].

© 1995 by The Haworth Press, Inc. All rights reserved.

no longer be thought of as hypochondriacs and that the Copenhagen Declaration will help them achieve their aims of disability awards (3).

I believe that the constellation of symptoms we now recognize is a reflection of an inability to cope, often because of patterns of behavior or expectation set up in childhood. As long as the rewards of this behavior pattern, provided by society, by doctors, etc., outweigh the debits, the pattern will be encouraged both at an individual and societal level. It is clear that FS patients do not fit into a single personality profile, and it remains possible or indeed likely that the syndrome may develop along various pathways, for example, borderline personality disorder, depression, or anxiety could all be predispositions. Furthermore, in some, the behavior pattern may develop in childhood as a result of deprivation or other forms of abuse. Our bodies send us a variety of sensations, most of which do not intrude on consciousness, but under some circumstances they may be noticed and taken as evidence of disease. Which symptoms we choose is influenced by fashion. Thus, given that patients are unquestionably convinced that they have organic disease, their symptoms will be governed unconsciously by what physicians can accept as being organic and by what the media may publicize. Even schizophrenic symptoms keep up with fashions and technical progress in a similar way. The WHO definition of health (4), "a state of complete physical, mental and social well-being and not merely the absence of disease or infirmity" may be part of the problem. By this definition most of us are not healthy. Studies of patients and control groups show a surprisingly high prevalence of various symptoms characteristic of FS when individuals are specifically asked for them. This is seen both in patients attending general medical clinics for other reasons (5) and in the general population (6,7).

I would like to review the history of some non-organic patterns of disease which may represent a "failure to cope" and may also represent what we now call fibromyalgia. These disorders have been expressed differently over the ages and the term "pathoplasticity" was coined by E. Shorter (8) to cover the changes in symptoms that are governed by fashions, both public and medical.

In the 16th and 17th centuries, demonic possession was not infrequent. I suspect few of us now consider this diagnosis. Not only is the diagnosis now rejected but the style of patient presentation with blasphemy, etc., leading to the diagnosis have disappeared. Why? Motor hysteria as described and codified by Charcot disappeared after Charcot's death. The description of the Babinsky response at this time led to a more reliable distinction between organic and non-organic paralyses. Therapeutic sympathy and interest then waned for those presentations that were evidently non-organic and new diseases developed. These syndromes are of course not all co-extensive and may differ significantly; but amongst many of them that I shall describe there appears to be a marked overlap.

Irritation in the spinal marrow was held to account for a "peculiar neuralgic affection of females" (9). In the UK in the 1840s a belief in widespread symptom production as a reflection of spinal abnormalities exceeds that of today's chiropractors. Brown-Sequard (10) later focused on the consequent irritation of centrepetal nerves, as a reflex representing disease of deeper organs.

A more pernicious doctrine was the connection of "insanity" with disease of the uterus (11) leading to mutilating surgery on the uterus, ovaries and clitoris. Eventually a controlled study (12) disproved the association but perhaps fashion also was working against it.

Alongside uterine explanations for disease developed neurasthenia. First described in 1869 (13), it was later described both as a fashionable new diagnosis and as an epidemic. Once again, as it gradually became accepted as non-organic in nature, a paradigm switch occurred. For treatment of diseases of the nervous system–"reflex abnormalities," "nervous exhaustion," "neurasthenia"–patients frequently visited "nerve doctors." As these physicians found more and more non-organic psychiatric aspects of disease, patients in their search for an organic explanation shifted to a different type of physician. It was recognized in the 1920s that the patient's presentation was unconsciously influenced by the doctor's expectations and theories.

Those physicians who recognized the non-organic nature of the problems bemoaned the fact that patients adamantly refused to accept this aspect, and this problem is echoed by subsequent generations over the years.

The term "shell shock" was coined during World War I to describe the cerebral symptoms that were sometimes experienced by soldiers in front line conditions. The term was acceptable as it was believed to represent an organic disorder of the brain akin to postconcussion syndromes related to the physical shock of a nearby explosion. After the psychiatric nature of the problem was eventually understood and the term no longer represented an organic disease with a definable external cause, the term fell largely into disuse.

Charts of 236 patients with a diagnosis of chronic nervous exhaustion were reviewed 6 years later by Macy et al. in 1934 from the Mayo Clinic (14). In virtually no cases had any new disease come to light to explain the previous findings. Like FS it was therefore a robust diagnostic category.

Other organic-sounding diagnoses have been used to cover the symptoms, so many of which are now described under fibromyalgia. Thus, chronic appendicitis was a frequent diagnosis for a brief period until surgical techniques allowed a demonstration of the error of this description. Similarly, chronic Brucellosis was an explanation for this constellation of symptoms. It never really gained wide acceptance and in the 1960s when serologic tests became available, the absence of previous exposure was demonstrable. The current counterpart is seen in today's Lyme disease diagnostic clinics where most of the patients attending with relevant symptoms cannot be shown to have had previous exposure to the spirochaete. Interestingly, the same problem is seen in lupus support groups–patients with vague symptoms looking for an organic diagnosis.

The "post-viral neurasthenia" perhaps began along with the LA polio epidemic in 1934. In 1984 the EBV link was constructed. When this was clearly shown to be untenable, it became chronic fatigue syndrome (15) and then chronic fatigue immunodeficiency syndrome. In the UK the processes were different and began in 1957 with the Royal Free disease (16). Although it was described in the original publication as a mysterious infection, others viewed it as a form of mass suggestibility. Follow up 25 years later showed that the problem persisted and behavioral explanations seemed likely (17). Out of this syndrome developed myalgic encephalomyelitis.

The relationship between these diagnoses–ME, neurasthenia, and others–is emphasized by Wessely (18). They are characterized by a presumption of organicity and a belief in an external causative factor. This applies especially to other recent diagnostic fashions such as chronic candidiasis, sick building syndrome, total environmental allergies, poisoning by mercury fillings, etc., and has been noted in chronic pain patients.

It is this presumption of organicity on the part of patients and physicians and the equally firm belief in an external causative factor that leads to the recurrent overinvestigation of our patients and their ever firmer, unconscious assumption of the "sick role" thrust on them by sympathetic physicians. It has also led to the appropriate array of research endeavors again to find an organic and etiologic explanation for the problems. Even the original observations of poor sleep patterns have been shown to be completely non-specific and seemingly therefore not of diagnostic importance (19,20). One of the frequent refrains of FS patients is how they can predict weather changes and how their symptoms become so much worse with certain types of change. This seemingly straightforward symptom is one that could be validated by experiment but when so assessed was found to be incorrect–an error of patient perception (21). While all symptoms are subjective–by definition–I believe the basis of the FS problem is the perception and distortion by consciousness of feelings normally ignored. The specific presentations relate to what doctors and patients expect (22). That these expectations change over the generations is described by the term "pathoplasticity," that is "the tendency of illness attribution and presentation to change with fashion" (8). Nowadays, these fashions rise and fall even more rapidly than before. This is spurred by sympathetic physicians, media attention, and to some degree patient support groups.

REFERENCES

1. Bennett RN: Disabling fibromyalgia: appearance versus reality. J Rheumatol 20:1821-1824, 1993.

2. Patrick DL, Deyo RA: Generic and disease specific measures in assessing health status and quality of life. Med Care 27:S217-S232, 1989.

3. Csillage C: Fibromyalgia: the Copenhagen Declaration. Lancet 340:663-664, 1992.

4. Basic Documents, 39th Edition. WHO, Geneva, 1992.

5. Campbell SM, Clark S, Tindall EA, Forehand ME, Bennett RM: Clinical characteristics of fibrositis. Arth & Rheum 26:817-824, 1983.

6. Croft P, Rigby AS, Boswell R, Schollum J, Silman A: The prevalence of chronic widespread pain in the population. J Rheum 20:710-713, 1993.

7. Forseth KD, Gram JT: The prevalence of fibromyalgia among women aged 20-49 years in Arendal, Norway. Scand J Rheum 21:74-78, 1992.

8. Shorter E: From paralysis to fatigue. McMillan Press, USA, 1992.

9. Parrish I: Remarks on spinal irritation as connected with nervous diseases. Amer J Mental Sciences 10:293-314, 1832.

10. Brown-Sequard E: Course of lectures on the physiology and pathology of the central nervous system. Lancet 2:519-520, 1858.

11. Wiglesworth J: On uterine disease and insanity. J Mental Science 30:509-531, 1885.

12. Dercum C: The nervous disorders in women simulating pelvic disease. Analysis of 591 cases. JAMA 52:848-851, 1909.

13. Beard G: Neurasthenia. Boston Med Surg J 80:217-221, 1869.

14. Macy JW, Allen EV: A justification for the diagnosis of chronic nervous exhaustion. Ann Int Med 7:861-867, 1934.

15. Holmes GP, Kaplan JE, et al: Chronic fatigue syndrome: a working case definition. Ann Int Med 108:387-389, 1988.

16. The Medical Staff of the Royal Free Hospital: An outbreak of encephalomyelitis in the Royal Free Hospital Group, London, in 1955. Brit Med J 2:895-904, 1957.

17. McEvedy CP, Beard AW: A controlled follow up of cases involved in an epidemic of "Benign myalgic encephalomyelitis." Br J Psych 122:141-150, 1973.

18. Wessely S: Old wine in new bottles: neurasthenia and "ME." Psycholog Med 20:35-53, 1990.

19. Hirsch M, et al: Objective and subjective sleep disturbances in patients with rheumatoid arthritis. Arth & Rheum 37:41-49, 1994.

20. Jennum P, Drewes AM, Andreasen A, Nielsen KD: Sleep and other symptoms in primary fibromyalgia and in healthy controls. J Rheum 20:1756-1759, 1993.

21. De Blecourt ACE, Kniping AA, De Voogd N, Van Rijswijk MH: Weather conditions and complaints in fibromyalgia. J Rheumatol 20:1932-1934, 1993.

22. Hadler N: Cumulative trauma disorder: an iatrogenic concept. J Occup Med 32:38-41, 1990.

Evidence for Abnormal Nociception in Fibromyalgia and Repetitive Strain Injury

Milton L. Cohen
Rachel B. Sheather-Reid
Jesus F. Arroyo
G. David Champion

SUMMARY. Objectives: To study psychophysical changes in fibromyalgia and "repetitive strain injury," respectively diffuse and regional cervicobrachial musculoskeletal pain syndromes. The clinical phenomena of tenderness [hyperalgesia] in particular but also dysesthesia, paresthesia and motor dysfunction occurring in the absence of tissue damage or disease suggest that altered nociception may be relevant to the pathogenesis of these disorders.

Methods: Non-noxious electrocutaneous stimulation in the upper limbs of patients with these syndromes was used as a psychophysical tool.

Results: No difference in the threshold for sensory perception but marked reduction in pain threshold and pain tolerance were found in

Milton L. Cohen, MB BS, MD, FRACP, is Staff Specialist in Rheumatology; Rachel B. Sheather-Reid, BSc (Hons), is Research Assistant; Jesus F. Arroyo, MD, FMH, is Research Fellow; and G. David Champion, MB BS, FRACP, is Consultant Rheumatologist, Department of Rheumatology, St. Vincent's Hospital, Sydney, NSW 2010, Australia.

Address correspondence to: Dr. Milton L. Cohen, Department of Rheumatology, St. Vincent's Hospital, Darlinghurst, NSW 2010, Australia.

[Haworth co-indexing entry note]: "Evidence for Abnormal Nociception in Fibromyalgia and Repetitive Strain Injury." Cohen, Milton L. et al. Co-published simultaneously in the *Journal of Musculoskeletal Pain* (The Haworth Medical Press, an imprint of The Haworth Press, Inc.) Vol. 3, No. 2, 1995, pp. 49-57; and: *Fibromyalgia, Chronic Fatigue Syndrome, and Repetitive Strain Injury: Current Concepts in Diagnosis, Management, Disability, and Health Economics* (ed: Andrew Chalmers et al.) The Haworth Medical Press, an imprint of The Haworth Press, Inc., 1995, pp. 49-57. Multiple copies of this article/chapter may be purchased from The Haworth Document Delivery Center [1-800-3-HA-WORTH; 9:00 a.m. - 5:00 p.m. (EST)].

© 1995 by The Haworth Press, Inc. All rights reserved.

patients compared with control subjects. Furthermore, the electrocu-taneous stimulation was accompanied by spread and persistence of dysesthesia, in painful limbs only.

Conclusion: These upper limbs were thus defined psychophysi-cally as well as clinically as regions of secondary hyperalgesia, which may imply that perturbation of central nociceptive mecha-nisms is involved in the pathogenesis of these syndromes.

KEYWORDS. Fibromyalgia, nociception, hyperalgesia, RSI, cu-mulative trauma disorder

INTRODUCTION

Fibromyalgia syndrome [FS] describes widespread musculoskeletal pain distinguished by the presence of "tender points," these forming the basis for the set of criteria proposed by the American College of Rheu-matology [ACR] (1). The construct of fibromyalgia as a distinct disease entity has been complicated by problems inherent in its circular argument, including the claim that it can coexist with any other condition (2). Despite extensive research efforts, no distinctive tissue pathology, pathophysiolo-gy or psychopathology has been found (3); in particular, the nature of the diagnostically mandatory "tender points" remains elusive.

Clinical features other than those in the ACR criteria have been men-tioned as part of the spectrum of FS, including subtle vasomotor distur-bances, altered cutaneous sensation, diffuse tenderness as well as the ten-der points, and worsening pain and hyperesthesia following clinical examination, defining hyperpathia (4,5).

Diffuse regional cervicobrachial pain [RCBP] associated with certain work tasks, although recognized since the 18th century, has appeared recently under a number of synonyms, including "occupational cervico-brachial disorder," "cumulative trauma disorder" and "repetitive strain injury" ["RSI"] (6). RCBP is a diagnostic label which is attached only after careful musculoskeletal and neurological examinations have failed to detect tissue damage or disease which can account for the associated clinical features. These include diffuse tenderness, cutaneous hypoesthe-sia, impairment of motor function and vasomotor and sudomotor distur-bances. Clinical examination in this syndrome also is commonly followed by hyperpathia (6).

Clinical Evidence for Altered Nociception

Thus, FS and RCBP share a number of clinical features. This has led to the proposal that RCBP [RSI] is a form of "localized FS," although that is unsatisfactory on epistemological grounds (6). The unifying clinical feature of both syndromes is tenderness or, more precisely, hyperalgesia, especially to mechanical stimulation, in deep musculoskeletal tissues. Hyperalgesia is defined as lowered threshold and increased response to noxious stimulation and operationally includes allodynia, pain in response to a non-noxious stimulus. Diagnostic reliance on tender points in fact depends upon elicitation of localized areas of clinical hyperalgesia. These clinical features can be articulated as clues to abnormal nociception [Table 1].

Psychophysical Evidence for Altered Nociception

Clinical psychophysics is an attempt to demonstrate quantitative relationships between subjective phenomena such as somatic sensations and the stimuli which elicit them. A variety of stimuli has been used in psychophysical studies: radiant heat, cold, mechanical, electrical, chemical and ischemic. The last two involve tissue injury, while the thermal techniques are not only dependent on vasomotor activity but also run the risk of tissue damage especially at tolerance levels. Mechanical techniques evoke both tactile and nociceptive responses. Electrocutaneous stimulation [ECS] elicits different qualities of pain than does thermal or mechanical stimulation and has the potential for activating all fiber types. This method may

TABLE 1. Inferences of abnormal nociception from clinical findings in FS and RCBP.

Clinical feature	Physiological inference
Hyperalgesia) Allodynia)	Sensitization of nociceptors, peripherally or centrally
Burning/electrical quality of pain	Coactivation of different fiber types
Hypoesthesia	Altered myelinated afferent function
Paresthesia/dysesthesia	Ectopic impulse formation
Local pain becoming diffuse	Receptive field enlargement
Hyperpathia	Consistent with known neuropathic pain states
Vasomotor and sudomotor changes	Sympathetic dysfunction
Dermatographia	Exaggerated axon reflex
Weakness without wasting	?Reflex ?antalgic ?dystonic

suffer least from method variance and has been validated in some pharmacological models for pain studies (8).

Both pain threshold and pain tolerance judgements need to be made in psychophysical studies of pain. These are not equivalent measures of responsiveness: the first emphasizes distinction of nociceptive quality, the second unwillingness to receive more intensive stimulation. Physiological and psychological factors affect these measures which are highly susceptible to placebo effect (8).

In FS, studies using pressure dolorimetry have identified mechanical hyperalgesia at both tender and non-tender points in FS patients compared with controls [summarized in (2) and (9)]. However this technique is limited by the difficulties of offering the stimulus randomly and of including supramaximal stimulation.

Following the observation that transcutaneous electrical nerve stimulation [TENS] frequently not only reproduced the pain but also evoked the paresthesia and dysesthesia of which patients with FS and RCBP complained, electrocutaneous stimulation [ECS] was used as an investigative psychophysical tool.

METHODS

Unidirectional square-wave pulses at 100Hz were delivered via silver electrodes to two specific test points on each upper limb, the palmar surfaces of the terminal phalanx of [1] the index finger and [2] the little finger, and to two points on the neck, 5 cm from the midline [3,4], selected to correspond to the dermatomes supplying limb sites [1] and [2], C5/6 and T1 respectively. Following familiarization during which they were not informed about characteristics of the stimulation or the nature of possible sensations, subjects were requested specifically to identify perception threshold [defined as minimally perceived sensation], pain threshold [when the sensation became unpleasant] and pain tolerance [defined as maximally tolerated unpleasant sensation and being signalled by a request for immediate cessation of stimulation or withdrawal of the arm].

Two test series were performed, using the ascending method of limits technique. In the first, a fixed pulse width of 60μsec was used with progressively increasing current [0-45mA] to determine perception threshold, pain threshold and pain tolerance. A second test series was then performed, recording pain threshold and pain tolerance only, using a constant current but increasing the pulse width of stimulus [40-1000 μsec]. For each individual the constant current used in this second test series had been determined in the first test series to produce a non-painful sensation similar to that at perception threshold. Each of the four test points was tested sequentially through the first and second series. This procedure was repeated three times at each site in random order.

RESULTS

Earlier Studies-FS [9] and RCBP [7]

In these studies perception threshold and pain tolerance only were measured. Control subjects were ten healthy volunteers [6 female; age range 19-40 years; all right-handed] who had no prior experience of chronic musculoskeletal pain. Ten patients with FS on the basis of the ACR criteria (1) were studied [8 female, age range 18-48 years, all right-handed]. Fifteen patients [14 female; age range 19-55 years; two left-handed] with well-established characteristic features of RCBP (6) were also tested. The affected side was in each case the dominant one; two patients had bilateral symptoms.

Perception threshold between FS and control subjects was similar. There was reduced pain tolerance in patients, both with increased current [arms] and increased pulse width [arms and necks]. ECS was associated with spread of sensation short of frank dysesthesia which persisted for up to 10 minutes. Perception threshold was similar between RCBP subjects and controls, as was pain tolerance when current was increased. However, when pulse width was increased, marked reduction in pain tolerance, associated with spread and persistence of dysesthesia, was reported by the RCBP patients but only on the affected side.

Later Studies

Using a more sophisticated ECS system, pain threshold as well as perception threshold and pain tolerance was studied. Ten naive patients with bilateral RCBP [who could also be labelled as FS except for their number of tender points] were tested: 8 female, age range 22-58 years. Eight healthy naive subjects [7 female, age range 25-45 years] were used as controls. Results are shown in Figure 1 [current variation] and Figure 2 [pulse width variation]. Perception threshold did not differ between patients and controls. Although there was a trend in patients towards lower pain threshold and pain tolerance with current variation, this reached statistical significance only in non-dominant limbs. However, when pulse width was increased, there was a trend towards lower pain threshold in both dominant and non-dominant limbs of patients, while the decrease in pain tolerance reached statistical significance. The difference between patients' pain threshold and pain tolerance in both stimulation series was narrow: the 95% confidence limits for that difference included zero. As before, ECS was associated with spread and persistence of dysesthesia but only in painful limbs.

DISCUSSION

As examples of clinical conditions characterized by diffuse musculo-skeletal pain in widespread or regional distribution, both FS (1) and RCBP (6) share clinical and psychophysical features which define the affected limbs as regions of secondary hyperalgesia (10).

Hyperalgesia [tenderness] occurring in undamaged tissue neurally related to a site of ongoing nociception is termed secondary. In contrast to primary hyperalgesia which is found in the zone of injury itself, regions of secondary hyperalgesia show normal threshold to potentially noxious stimulation as well as, by definition, decreased tolerance to mechanical and thermal stimuli. Electrocutaneous stimulation in FS and RCBP revealed normal perception threshold and reduced pain tolerance, features which strongly resemble the responses to mechanical stimulation.

The principal neural mechanism in secondary hyperalgesia is considered to involve changed excitability of spinal cord neurons and is most dependent on the activity of unmyelinated or small myelinated primary afferents (10,11). The present results, with respect to both threshold and tolerance measures and the phenomena of spread and persistence of dysesthesia, are consistent with a state of activation and sensitization of specific nociceptive afferents. It is also possible that non-nociceptive A fibers may be mechanistically responsible for the phenomena reported, again as a likely result of changed central processing (11). Factors inducing this plasticity in the spinal cord include persistent nociceptive input, which may be relevant to the pathogenesis of FS and RCBP (6,9,12).

The clinically provokable hyperesthetic signs in these two chronic musculoskeletal pain syndromes, taken together with the psychophysical demonstration of normal perception threshold, lowered pain threshold and reduced pain tolerance, suggest that the relevant pathophysiological mechanism is that of secondary hyperalgesia. In turn, this implies that enhanced nociception, probably at a spinal cord level, is the somatic contribution to chronicity of these syndromes in which the roles of cognitive, affective and behavioral factors must also be considered.

FIGURE 1. Perception threshold, pain threshold and pain tolerance in response to increasing current [mA] at constant pulse width. Open columns: control subjects [CONTROL]; filled columns: patients with bilateral RCBP [BILATERAL]. Upper panel: dominant limbs [DOM]; lower panel: non-dominant limbs [NDOM]. Means and 95% confidence intervals shown. *P < 0.05.

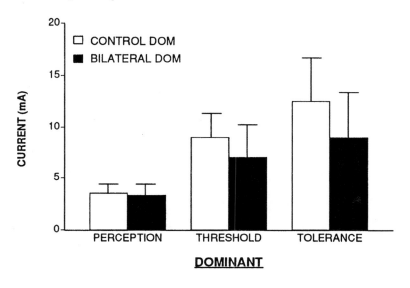

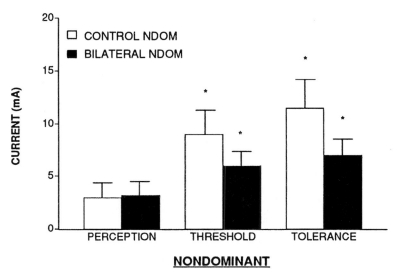

FIGURE 2. Pain threshold and pain tolerance in response to increasing pulse width [μsec] at constant current. Perception threshold already exceeded. Open hatched columns: control subjects [CONTROL]; filled hatched columns: patients with bilateral RCBP [BILATERAL]. Upper panel: dominant limbs [DOM]; lower panel: non-dominant limbs [NDOM]. Means and 95% confidence intervals shown. *P < 0.05.

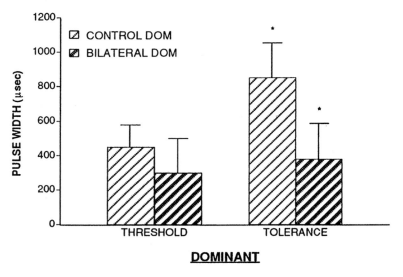

DOMINANT

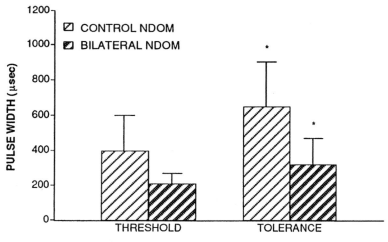

NONDOMINANT

REFERENCES

1. Wolfe F, Smythe HA, Yunus MB, Bennett RM, Bombardier C, Goldenberg DL, Tugwell P, Campbell SM, Abeles M, Clark P, Fam AG, Farber SJ, Fiechtner JJ, Franklin CM, Gatter RA, Hamaty D, Lessard J, Lichtbroun AS, Masi AT, McCain GA, Reynolds WJ, Romano TJ, Russell IJ, Sheon RP: The American College of Rheumatology 1990 Criteria for the classification of fibromyalgia. Arthritis Rheum 33:160-173, 1990.

2. Cohen ML, Quintner JL: Fibromyalgia syndrome–a problem of tautology. Lancet 342:906-909, 1993.

3. Boissevan MD, McCain GA: Towards an integrated understanding of fibromyalgia syndrome. Pain 45:227-238 & 239-248, 1991.

4. Simms RW, Goldenberg DL: Symptoms mimicking neurologic disorders in Fibromyalgia Syndrome. J Rheumatol 15:1271-1273, 1988.

5. Quimby LG, Block SR, Gratwick GM: Fibromyalgia: generalized pain intolerance and manifold symptom reporting. J Rheumatol 15:1264-70, 1988.

6. Cohen ML, Arroyo JF, Champion GD, Browne CD: In search of the pathogenesis of refractory cervicobrachial pain syndrome: a deconstruction of the RSI phenomenon. Med J Aust 156:432-436, 1992.

7. Arroyo JF, Cohen ML: Unusual responses to electrocutaneous stimulation in refractory cervicobrachial pain: clues to a neuropathic pathogenesis. Clin Exp Rheumatol 10:475-482, 1992.

8. Harris G, Rollman GB: The validity of experimental pain measures. Pain 17:369-376, 1983.

9. Arroyo JF, Cohen ML: Abnormal responses to electrocutaneous stimulation in fibromyalgia. J Rheumatol 20:1925-31, 1993.

10. Treede R-D, Meyer RA, Raja SN, Campbell JN: Peripheral and central mechanisms of cutaneous hyperalgesia. Progr Neurobiol 38:397-421, 1992.

11. Dubner R: Neuronal plasticity and pain following peripheral tissue inflammation or nerve injury, Proceedings of the VIth World Congress on Pain. Edited by MR Bond, JE Charlton & CJ Woolf. Elsevier, Amsterdam, 1991, pp. 263-276.

12. Gracely RH, Lynch S, Bennett GB: Painful neuropathy: altered central processing maintained dynamically by peripheral input. Pain 51:175-194, 1992.

Neurohormonal:
Abnormal Laboratory Findings Related
to Pain and Fatigue in Fibromyalgia

I. Jon Russell

KEYWORDS. Fibromyalgia, pathogenesis, serotonin, substance P, allodynia

INTRODUCTION

Fibromyalgia syndrome [FS] is a chronic, painful, musculoskeletal disorder of unknown etiology. For many years, the problem was thought to reside in the skeletal muscles near where the pain was experienced, but careful histological study has failed to identify a specific structural abnormality. Those revelations have provided support for a *metabolic* pathogenesis. The diffuse nature of the disorder, involving pain in a variety of types of soft tissue, has led to the hypothesis that the pain in FS has its origin in the central nervous system [CNS].

One or more metabolic or neurotransmitter abnormalities could cause interpretive defects in the CNS function capable of distorting the patient's

---

I. Jon Russell, MD, PhD, is affiliated with the Department of Medicine, University of Texas Health Science Center, San Antonio, TX.

Address correspondence to: I. Jon Russell, MD, PhD, Department of Medicine, Division of Clinical Immunology, University of Texas Health Science Center, 7703 Floyd Curl Drive, San Antonio, TX 78284-7874.

[Haworth co-indexing entry note]: "Neurohormonal: Abnormal Laboratory Findings Related to Pain and Fatigue in Fibromyalgia." Russell, I. Jon. Co-published simultaneously in the *Journal of Musculoskeletal Pain* (The Haworth Medical Press, an imprint of The Haworth Press, Inc.) Vol. 3, No. 2, 1995, pp. 59-65; and: *Fibromyalgia, Chronic Fatigue Syndrome, and Repetitive Strain Injury: Current Concepts in Diagnosis, Management, Disability, and Health Economics* (ed: Andrew Chalmers et al.) The Haworth Medical Press, an imprint of The Haworth Press, Inc., 1995, pp. 59-65. Multiple copies of this article/chapter may be purchased from The Haworth Document Delivery Center [1-800-3-HAWORTH; 9:00 a.m. - 5:00 p.m. (EST)].

© 1995 by The Haworth Press, Inc. All rights reserved.

perception of pain in the absence of peripheral tissue injury. That concept prompted us to view FS as a form of "chronic widespread allodynia," a perception of pain resulting from normal stimuli. On this basis, the arena in which to seek information about the pathogenesis of FS has changed. It also provides an explanation for neuroendocrine abnormalities in FS.

HYPOTHALAMIC-PITUITARY-ADRENAL [HPA] AXIS

Fatigue and depression in FS prompted a series of HPA assessments. They revealed a number of abnormalities which will have to be accommodated in any pathogenic explanation of FS.

FS patients exhibited an abnormal diurnal pattern in plasma cortisol levels and decreased 24 hour excretion of cortisol (1). The secretion of ACTH in response to CRH was abnormally exuberant in FS suggesting a lack of feedback regulation by cortisol (2). Since cortisol production in those settings was inappropriately low relative to the ACTH surge, it seemed likely that a "lethargic" adrenal might be partially at fault for both phenomena.

Another aspect of hypothalamic-pituitary dysfunction in FS involves the secretion of human growth hormone [HGH] during deep sleep. Poor sleep in FS results in a deficiency in HGH which then fails to induce normal production of IGF1 by the liver (3). Our laboratory has confirmed that finding and shown that dehydroepiandrosterone sulfate [DHEAS], an adrenal steroid partially regulated by IGF1, is also low in FS sera. By analogy to the HPA axis, this system involving HGH, IGF1 and DHEAS could be referred to as the hypothalamic-pituitary-liver-adrenal [HPLA] axis.

Prolactin is another pituitary product which is frequently elevated in the blood of endocrinology clinic patients with galactorrhea. The prevalence of FS in affected individuals may be as high as 70% (4). In our rheumatology practice, galactorrhea has been rare [< 1%] in FS patients and our laboratory assessment has indicated normal serum prolactin levels. Therefore, prolactin excess alone is not necessary for the development of FS.

SUBSTANCE P [SP]

Substance P [SP] is one of several neuropeptides which are involved in the process of nociception (5). A study conducted in Norway (6) found SP to be 3-fold elevated in cerebrospinal fluid [CSF] of FS patients compared with control subjects but did not document its relationship to the FS symptoms. A similar study was conducted by our group with CSF from 32 FS patients and 30 healthy normal controls [NC]. The FS patients were significantly older and included a higher proportion of females than the NC. Our findings were very similar to those previously reported, with 42.8 ± 14.9 fmole/ml in FS CSF versus 16.3 ± 6.04 in NC CSF [P < 0.001]. Age and gender had no influence on CSF SP levels. As dramatic as the differences in CSF SP were between FS patients and NC subjects, its correlation [R = −0.30] in FS patients with the clinical severity of the painful symptoms was weak. These data suggest that the elevated SP levels in FS patients are probably related to the pathogenesis of the pain, but that it is not acting alone. As earlier predicted (7), a likely candidate for the pivotal "other abnormality" would be inadequate 5HT effect.

SEROTONIN [5HT]

The metabolic precursor of 5HT is tryptophan [TRP], an essential amino acid which humans must acquire from their diet. Our initial study demonstrated TRP to be significantly [P = 0.002] lower than normal in the sera of FS patients (8) but 6 other amino acids [alanine, histidine, lysine, proline, serine, and threonine] were also low. The report of Yunus et al. (9) supported these findings and disclosed a defect in the transport of TRP across cell membranes.

The mechanism responsible for the low TRP is not known, but one possibility was a diversion of TRP into the kynurenine [KYN] pathway. The enzyme tryptophan-2,3-dioxygenase converts TRP to KYN which is then converted to 3-hydroxykynurenine [3HKY]. We measured KYN in the sera of FS patients and NC subjects but found only small, non-significant differences between the 2 groups. It was interesting, however, that the serum KYN correlated inversely with serum 5HT [R = −0.62, P < 0.0001] and weakly with the FS patients' perception of pain [Visual Analog Scale, R = 0.35, P = 0.03].

The situation was different in the cerebrospinal fluid [CSF] of FS patients, where we found the concentration of KYN to be significantly [P = 0.03] higher and the next metabolite, 3HKY, to be 50% lower than normal. The increased KYN concentration, in the setting of a borderline low CSF TRP, indicated an increased CNS activity of the enzyme indole-2,3-dioxygenase [IDO]. The decreased 3HKY indicated lower than normal activity of kynurenine-3-oxygenase [K3O] which depends upon NADP as a cofactor.

We then measured adenine nucleotides in the red blood cells [RBC] of 28 FS patients compared with those of 28 matched NC subjects, and found significantly lower than normal RBC NADP [P = 0.05], NADH [P = 0.024], and ATP [P < 0.006]. NADP in the FS patients' RBC correlated highly with RBC ATP [R = 0.73, P < 0.001], an association not present in NC subjects' RBC. However, none of the nucleotide levels correlated with the FS perception of pain, or fatigue. These findings from 2 different compartments support the possibility that K3O activity may be diminished because of an NADP deficiency in FS.

It is of interest that interferon is known to enhance the activity of IDO and to induce the polymerization of NADP resulting in a depletion of its cellular stores (10). We currently are attempting to determine whether there are increased levels of interferon in FS CSF.

Our laboratory also examined the concentration of 5HT in patients' sera and found significantly decreased levels in FS patients compared with matched NC (11). Those results have now been confirmed by 2 separate studies, one from our laboratory and another from a Swiss group (12). The later study also reported that the serum 5HT levels in FS patients correlated with the severity of perceived pain, but we have been unable to confirm that association.

It was assumed that the source of the 5HT in sera was circulating platelets which could variably release 5HT when activated by the clotting process. An experiment just completed in our laboratory has shown that washed platelets from FS patients did indeed contain significantly less 5HT than NC. Among FS patients, a correlation was found between the platelet 5HT and the number of tender points by dolorimetry examination, so it appears that platelet 5HT is related to the painful symptoms of FS. That finding of low intra-platelet 5HT in FS was consistent with our earlier report (11) of higher than normal numbers of 5HT re-uptake [^{3}H-imipramine binding] receptors on the surfaces of peripheral platelets in FS, suggesting a servo-mechanism response to inadequate intra-platelet 5HT. The relationship between low platelet 5HT and the report of anti-5HT antibodies in FS (13) is unknown.

Our prior study (14) of CSF from FS patients had indicated that 5-hydroxyindole acetic acid [5HIAA], the immediate product of 5HT metabolism is numerically but not significantly low in FS.

5HT REGULATION OF HPA AND HPLA

Evidence from animal models has indicated that activation of 5HT and norepinephrine receptors regulate the HPA axis (15). 5HT receptor mechanisms control the synthesis of corticotrophin releasing hormone [CRH], which stimulates the pituitary to produce adrenal corticotrophin [ACTH].

The abnormalities in the function of HPA and HPLA axes in FS are consistent with alterations in 5HT receptor activation.

5HT REGULATION OF SP

Experiments using a rat model have shown that the nociceptive effects of SP in the spinal cord are counteracted by 5HT agonists (16). On the other hand, 5HT appears to up-regulate SP synthesis in the rat brain (17). It is curious that parachlorophenylalanine [PCPA, blocks 5HT production] treatment of whole rat brain reduced brain SP levels by 87% while at the same time increasing the spinal cord SP content by over 100% (18). These data indicate an inverse relationship between brain SP and spinal cord SP concentrations. In addition, rat brain SP seems to function as a central down-regulator of nociception by increasing cord level 5HT. If these data from rat experiments are applicable to the human system, one would expect low CNS 5HT and SP, high spinal cord SP but low spinal cord 5HT in FS.

WORKING MODEL

Our simplest model to explain these findings focuses on a decrease in 5HT effect [failure to properly activate 5HT receptors] on 5HT regulated systems in the CNS. It would appear that a decrease in 5HT effect can cause each of the following: decreases in HPA hormone production, delta wave sleep, HPLA hormone production, brain SP, and spinal cord 5HT; increases in spinal cord SP; and chronic diffuse allodynia.

We are currently unaware of any clinical findings or laboratory data which would specifically invalidate this model but it doesn't yet have a satisfying starting point. What could cause the low 5HT effect? Is it due to a CNS deficiency of 5HT, a 5HT inhibitor, an anti-5HT antibody, a defective 5HT receptor? If a 5HT deficiency is implicated, is it due to an excess of IFN, due perhaps to a viral infection or some other mechanism?

REFERENCES

1. Crofford LJ, Pillemer SR, Kalogeras KT, Cash JM, Michelson D, King MA, Sternberg EM, Gold PW, Chrousos GP, Wilder RL: Perturbations of hypothalamic-pituitary-adrenal axis function in patients with fibromyalgia. Arthritis Rheum 36(9):S220, 1993.

2. Griep EN, Boersma JW, deKloet ER: Altered reactivity of the hypothalamic-pituitary-adrenal axis in the primary fibromyalgia syndrome. J Rheumatol 20:469-474, 1993.

3. Bennett RM, Clark SR, Campbell SM, Burckhardt CS: Low levels of somatomedin C in patients with the fibromyalgia syndrome: A possible link between sleep and muscle pain. Arthritis Rheum 35:1113-1116, 1992.

4. Buskila D, Fefer P, Harman-Boehm I, Press J, Neumann L, Gedalia A, Sukenik S: Assessment of nonarticular tenderness and prevalence of fibromyalgia in hyperprolactinemic women. Arthritis Rheum 35(Suppl):S114, 1992.

5. Maimberg AB, Yaksh TL: Hyperalgesia mediated by spinal glutamate or substance P receptor blocked by spinal cyclooxygenase inhibition. Science 257:1276-1279, 1992.

6. Vaeroy H, Helle R, Forre O, Kass E, Terenius L: Elevated CSF levels of substance P and high incidence of Raynaud's phenomenon in patients with fibromyalgia: New features for diagnosis. Pain 32:21-26,1988.

7. Russell IJ: Neurohormonal aspects of fibromyalgia syndrome. In: Rheumatic Disease Clinics of North America. Edited by RM Bennett and DL Goldenberg. W.B. Saunders, Philadelphia, 1989, pp. 149-168.

8. Russell IJ, Michalek JE, Vipraio GA, Fletcher EM, Wall K: Serum amino acids in fibrositis/fibromyalgia syndrome. J Rheumatol 19:158-163,1989.

9. Yunus MB, Dailey JW, Aldag JC, Masi AT, Jobe PC: Plasma tryptophan and other amino acids in primary fibromyalgia: A controlled study. J Rheumatol 19:90-94, 1992.

10. Aune TM, Pogue SL: Inhibition of tumor cell growth by interferon-gamma is mediated by two distinct mechanisms dependent upon oxygen tension: Induction of tryptophan degradation and depletion of intracellular nicotinamide adenine dinucleotide. Journal of Clinical Investigation 84:863-875, 1989.

11. Russell IJ, Michalek JE, Vipraio GA, Fletcher EM, Javors MA, Bowden CA: Platelet 3H-imipramine uptake receptor density and serum serotonin levels in patients with fibromyalgia/fibrositis syndrome. J Rheumatol 19:104-109, 1992.

12. Hrycaj P, Stratz T, Muller W: Platelet ^{3}H-imipramine uptake receptor density and serum serotonin in patients with fibromyalgia/fibrositis syndrome. J Rheumatol 20:1986-1987, 1993.

13. Klein R, Bansch M, Berg PA: Clinical relevance of antibodies against serotonin and gangliosides in patients with primary fibromyalgia syndrome. Psycho-Neuro-Endocrinol 17:593-598, 1992.

14. Russell IJ, Vaeroy H, Javors M, Nyberg F: Cerebrospinal fluid biogenic amine metabolites in fibromyalgia/fibrositis syndrome and rheumatoid arthritis. Arthritis Rheum 35:550-556, 1992.

15. Burnet PWJ, Mefford IN, Smith CC, Gold PW, Sternberg EM: Hippocampal 8-[3H]hydroxy-2-(di-n-propylamino)tetralin binding site densities, serotonin receptor (5HT1A) messenger ribonucleic acid abundance, and serotonin levels parallel the activity of the hypothalamopituitary-adrenal axis in rat. J Neurochem 59:1062-1070, 1992.

16. Eide PK, Hole K: Interactions between serotonin and substance P in the spinal regulation of nociception. Brain Research 550:225-230,1991.

17. Walker PD, Riley LA, Hart RP, Jonakait GM: Serotonin regulation of ta-chykinin biosynthesis in the rat neostriatum. Brain Research 546:33-39,1991.

18. Sharma HS, Nyberg F, Olsson Y, Dey PK: Alteration of substance P after trauma to the spinal cord: An experimental study in the rat. Neuroscience 38:205-212, 1990.

Hypothalamic-Pituitary-Adrenal Axis Dysregulation in Fibromyalgia and Chronic Fatigue Syndrome: An Overview and Hypothesis

Mark A. Demitrack
Leslie J. Crofford

INTRODUCTION

Our group has suggested that the mutually exclusive distinction implied by the strictly "psychological" and "physiological" etiologies proposed for fibromyalgia syndrome [FS] and chronic fatigue syndrome [CFS] may be more apparent than real. We proposed that the phenomenologic overlap between FS and CFS and a variety of primary psychiatric illnesses may reflect the involvement of a shared, biological pathway that may be similarly dysregulated by a disparate variety of infectious or non-infectious antecedent events. Considered from this perspective, several issues would suggest that a focus on the hypothalamic-pituitary-adrenal [HPA] axis is a

Mark A. Demitrack, MD, is affiliated with the Department of Psychiatry, University of Michigan Medical Center, Ann Arbor, MI. Leslie J. Crofford, MD, is affiliated with the Department of Internal Medicine, University of Michigan Medical Center, Ann Arbor, MI.

Address correspondence to: Mark A. Demitrack, MD, Department of Psychiatry, University of Michigan Medical Center, 1500 East Medical Center Drive, Ann Arbor, MI 48109-0118.

[Haworth co-indexing entry note]: "Hypothalamic-Pituitary-Adrenal Axis Dysregulation in Fibromyalgia and Chronic Fatigue Syndrome: An Overview and Hypothesis." Demitrack, Mark A., and Leslie J. Crofford. Co-published simultaneously in the *Journal of Musculoskeletal Pain* (The Haworth Medical Press, an imprint of The Haworth Press, Inc.) Vol. 3, No. 2, 1995, pp. 67-73; and: *Fibromyalgia, Chronic Fatigue Syndrome, and Repetitive Strain Injury: Current Concepts in Diagnosis, Management, Disability, and Health Economics* (ed: Andrew Chalmers et al.) The Haworth Medical Press, an imprint of The Haworth Press, Inc., 1995, pp. 67-73. Multiple copies of this article/chapter may be purchased from The Haworth Document Delivery Center [1-800-3-HAWORTH; 9:00 a.m. - 5:00 p.m. (EST)].

© 1995 by The Haworth Press, Inc. All rights reserved.

particularly useful domain of study and may help in establishing a more integrative view of the pathophysiology of these syndromes.

It is a frequent clinical observation that patients with FS and CFS often report the onset of their illness following a significant period of stress [e.g., accidental trauma, infection, emotional stress, overwork, sleep disruption], and that the course of the syndrome waxes and wanes with subsequent periods of physical or emotional stress. The HPA axis is generally considered to be the prototypical hormonal stress system of the body. Regulation of this system involves a complex array of biochemical events coordinating the activities of the hypothalamus, the pituitary, and the adrenal gland. Suprahypothalamic influences such as the brainstem catecholamine system serve as important "activation" pathways for this system during stress. In addition to these stress-dependent activational pathways, intrinsic rhythmic elements in the suprachiasmatic nucleus drive the HPA axis in a circadian fashion. In humans, the circadian rhythm of ACTH and cortisol secretion is entrained to the sleep/wake cycle, with the trough of activity occurring in the evening and early night, and the peak in activity occurring just before waking.

A seminal observation heralding the era of biological psychiatry was that patients with major depression demonstrated a characteristic disruption of the normal diurnal rhythm of the HPA axis. This disturbance involves an elevation of circulating glucocorticoids, with an earlier onset of the morning surge of the axis, in conjunction with enhanced cortisol secretion in the late afternoon. More recently, detailed studies of the HPA axis have refined our understanding of the biochemical events responsible for this finding. A model of HPA axis dysregulation has been developed on the basis of this work, suggesting that in some forms of major depression, there is an excessive central release of the hypothalamic-releasing hormone, CRH, with the subsequent development of adrenal gland hypertrophy due to chronic overstimulation of the target organ itself.

Despite this observation, it has become apparent that depression is a heterogeneous condition from both a psychological and a physiological perspective. The initial investigations of the neuroendocrine correlates of depression largely concerned the more classical, melancholic form of depression, namely that characterized by increased agitation, loss of sleep, loss of interest in all activities, persistent suicidal thoughts, and reduced appetite and libido. More recently, several alternate forms of depressive illness have been described which lack the typical features of melancholic depression. These depressive subtypes are of particular interest because of their overlap with the symptoms of FS and CFS. They are usually dominated by reduced energy, a reactive mood and a reversal of the typical pattern of vegetative features seen in classical depression. Examples of these syndromes include the depressive phase of manic-depressive illness, seasonal affective disorder, "atypical" major depression, and the depressive syndromes seen in the context of certain endocrinopathies such as primary hypothyroidism and the post-operative state of Cushing's disease. Recent evidence suggests a pattern of HPA function in some of these syndromes reflecting inappropriately normal or frankly reduced activation of the axis. It has been suggested that the unifying feature of the HPA axis disturbance associated with these conditions is a functional *deficit* in the release of hypothalamic CRH. This is of interest since CRH serves not only as a principal stimulus to the HPA axis, but also because it is a behaviorally-active neurohormone whose central administration to animals and non-human primates induces signs of physiological and behavioral arousal. Hence, a relative or absolute deficiency of hypothalamic CRH could contribute to the profound lethargy and fatigue that are inherent characteristics of these "atypical" depressive syndromes, FS, and/or CFS, either through direct effects upon the central nervous system or indirectly by causing a relative glucocorticoid deficiency.

Could a relative glucocorticoid deficiency itself contribute to the observed symptoms of "atypical" depressive syndromes, FS, and/or CFS? A review of the clinical features of these illnesses shows considerable overlap with the symptoms seen in patients with glucocorticoid deficiency. Indeed, one of the principal symptoms of glucocorticoid deficiency is debilitating fatigue. An abrupt onset precipitated by a stressor, arthralgias, myalgias, feverishness, adenopathy, post-exertional fatigue, exacerbation of allergic responses, and disturbances in mood and sleep are also characteristic of glucocorticoid insufficiency. Furthermore, since glucocorticoids are the most potent endogenous immunosuppressive compounds, we also suggest that some of the reported immunologic disturbances in patients with FS or CFS may also reflect the immune activation that might be expected to accompany a mild or relative glucocorticoid deficiency. In this regard, it has been shown, in animals, that a defect in the responsiveness of the HPA axis to immune mediators confers a risk for the development of inflammatory disease (1). Furthermore, in humans, withdrawal from hypercortisolemic states has been associated with the exacerbation of autoimmune thyroiditis (2), as well as the development of myalgias, arthralgias, muscle weakness (3), and even severe FS (4).

The phenomenologic similarity of FS and CFS with some forms of depression, in addition to the biochemical considerations outlined above, lend further interest toward an examination of the specific neuroendocrine characteristics of patients with FS and CFS. Several studies add to this interest. For example, McCain and Tilbe reported that patients with FS have reduced 24-hour urine free cortisol excretion and a loss of the diurnal fluctuation of glucocorticoid levels (5). More recently, Griep and colleagues reported exaggerated ACTH, but blunted cortisol response to exogenous administration of CRH and to insulin-induced hypoglycemia (6). These latter 2 studies of HPA axis function in FS are remarkably similar to the data we have reported (7,8), and lend further support to the hypothesis of HPA axis dysfunction as a reproducible biologic correlate of FS.

HPA AXIS DYSREGULATION IN FS AND CFS: AN HYPOTHESIS

Taken together, our data and the work of others suggest that a unifying characteristic of HPA axis function in FS and CFS is a moderate basal hypocortisolism, as reflected by a reduction in the 24-hour excretion of urine free cortisol. These observations stand in sharp contrast with the glucocorticoid excess seen in classical, melancholic depression. Despite this apparent similarity in overall adrenocortical function, closer observation reveals distinct, and sometimes divergent, HPA axis findings in FS and CFS. These observations are summarized in Table 1.

Several different disruptions in the integrated function of the HPA axis may underlie these abnormalities. A deficit in maximal adrenal responsiveness is clearly present in both illnesses, however, this finding is unlikely to serve as the primary and sole explanation for the collection of

TABLE 1. Summary of Principal HPA Axis Findings in Patients with FS and CFS.

		Fibromyalgia Syndrome	Chronic Fatigue Syndrome
BRAIN	• Insulin tolerance testing	Impaired	---------
	• CSF CRH, ACTH	---------	?Reduced
	• Diurnal rhythm	Blunted	---------
PITUITARY	• Basal PM ACTH	Normal	Elevated
	• oCRH challenge	Exaggerated	Blunted
ADRENAL	• Basal PM cortisol	Elevated	Reduced
	• 24-Hour UFC	Reduced	Reduced
	• ACTH challenge	---------	↑sensitivity, ↓capacity
	• oCRH challenge	Reduced	Normal

findings we have reported. Indeed, the weight of available data would suggest that the impaired adrenal reserve is a late finding, evolving as a result of chronic understimulation of the gland itself. What are the possible mechanisms of the understimulation of the adrenal? Several potential mechanisms are outlined in Table 2. An alteration in pituitary function is an intriguing possibility. Indeed, the observation of exaggerated ACTH release in FS may be explained by an increased pituitary content of the immediate releasable pool of POMC-derived peptides. Such a phenomenon is seen in animals during chronic stress, where the anterior pituitary content of ACTH increases. However, this implies persistent central activation of the HPA axis, due either to increased activity of CRH itself, or the neural or biochemical circuits impinging upon CRH secretion. Elsewhere we have argued that, as a whole, the observations of HPA axis function in FS and CFS are *not* similar to the findings in stress-related illnesses presumed to be associated with increased CRH activity [e.g., melancholic depression], though this possibility cannot be entirely ruled out from the data we have assembled.

Enhanced ACTH release may also emerge from two other considerations: an increase in the number or sensitivity of pituitary CRH receptors, or an increased activity of other ACTH secretagogues. Pituitary ACTH responsiveness during stress is determined in large part by the combined activity of both CRH and the other principal stress-related secretagogue, arginine vasopressin [AVP], which acts in synergy with CRH to stimulate synthesis and release of ACTH from the anterior pituitary. If, as suggested by our preliminary data, AVP levels are increased in patients with FS, one would expect increased ACTH secretion in response to exogenous CRH. Interestingly, Behan and colleagues have reported *reduced* AVP levels in response to fluid restriction in patients with CFS (9). Hence, low AVP levels in patients with CFS could explain some of the differences between CFS and FS seen during stimulatory testing of the HPA axis. It should be emphasized that these measurements of circulating AVP reflect activity of

TABLE 2. Hypothetical Factors That May Contribute to Impaired HPA Axis Activation in FS and CFS.

- Primary defect in adrenal responsiveness
- Altered pituitary sensitivity
- Altered hypothalamic drive
- Disruption in suprahypothalamic influences on the axis [neural, biochemical]
- Altered circadian rhythm
- Increased sensitivity to glucocorticoid negative feedback

magnocellular AVP, which may not be a true reflection of the activity of the parvocellular sources of AVP.

Might the understimulation of adrenal function emerge from an even more centrally-located disruption in the HPA axis than just the pituitary? A potential answer to this question is suggested by several recent animal models characterized by impaired activation of the HPA axis due to an apparent reduction in hypothalamic CRH secretion. For example, in the Piebald-Viral-Glaxo rat strain during the development of mycobacterially-induced adjuvant arthritis, there is an increase in anterior pituitary POMC mRNA, however, a marked *reduction* in the synthesis and release of hypothalamic CRH mRNA in the PVN is observed at the same time (10). Coincident with this fall in CRH is an increase in the level of AVP in the hypophyseal portal system. Another animal model for hypothalamic CRH hypofunction, the Lewis rat, exhibits an impaired activation of the HPA axis in response to inflammatory and non-inflammatory stressors (1). These blunted HPA axis responses are associated with deficient hypothalamic CRH expression in comparison with the histocompatible Fisher rats. However, Lewis rats also exhibit markedly elevated plasma and hypothalamic AVP levels compared with Fisher rats (11). Finally, an even more intriguing observation that is not restricted to a specific rat strain type, is the impaired HPA axis activation seen in the acute stress model of cholestasis due to bile duct resection (12). In these animals, a reduction of hypothalamic CRH synthesis is seen, in conjunction with a dramatic rise in hypothalamic AVP. Some aspects of these animal models bear a similarity to the neuroendocrine characteristics of patients with FS and CFS.

In summary, it appears that reduced adrenal glucocorticoid secretion serves as a common feature of CFS and FS. However, our data and the work of others suggest that there may be differing patterns of dysregulation in the separate components of the HPA axis in patients with FM and CFS.

REFERENCES

1. Sternberg EM, Hill JM, Chrousos GP, Kamilaris T, Listwak SJ, Gold PW, Wilder RL: Inflammatory Mediator-Induced Hypothalamic-Pituitary-Adrenal Activation is Defective in Streptococcal Cell Wall Arthritis-Susceptible Rats. Proc Natl Acad Sci USA 1989; 86:2374-2378.

2. Takasu N, Komiya I, Nagasawa Y, Asawa T, Yamada T: Exacerbation of Autoimmune Thyroid Dysfunction After Unilateral Adrenalectomy in Patients with Cushing's Syndrome due to an Adrenocortical Adenoma. N Engl J Med 1990; 322(24):1708-1712.

3. Dixon RB, Christy NP: On the Various Forms of Corticosteroid Withdrawal Syndrome. Am J Med 1980; 68(2):224-230.

4. Disdier P, Harle J-R, Brue T, Jaquet P, Chambourlier P, Grisoll F, Weiller P-J: Severe Fibromyalgia After Hypophysectomy for Cushing's Disease. Arthr and Rheum 1991; 34(4):493-495.

5. McGain GA, Tilbe KS: Diurnal Hormone Variation in Fibromyalgia Syndrome: A Comparison with Rheumatoid Arthritis. J Rheumatol 1989 [suppl]; 16:154-157.

6. Griep EN, Boersma JW, deKloet ER: Altered Reactivity of the Hypothalamic-Pituitary-Adrenal Axis in the Primary Fibromyalgia Syndrome. J Rheumatol 1993; 20:469-474.

7. Demitrack MA, Dale JK, Straus SE, Laue L, Listwak SJ, Kruesi MJP, Chrousos GP, Gold PW: Evidence for Impaired Activation of the Hypothalamic-Pituitary-Adrenal Axis in Patients with Chronic Fatigue Syndrome. J Clin Endo Metab 1991; 73(6):1224-1234.

8. Crofford LJ, Pillemer SR, Kalogeras KT, Cash JM, Michelson D, Kling MA, Sternberg EM, Gold PW, Chrousos GP, Wilder RL: Hypothalamic-Pituitary-Adrenal Axis Perturbations in Patients with Fibromyalgia, Rheumatol, in press.

9. Bakheit AMO, Behan PO, Watson WS, Morton JJ: Abnormal Arginine Vasopressin Secretion and Water Metabolism in Patients with Postviral Fatigue Syndrome. Acta Neurol Scand 1993; 87:234-238.

10. Harbuz MS, Rees RG, Eckland D, Jessop DS, Brewerton D, Lightman SL: Paradoxical Responses of Hypothalamic Corticotropin-Releasing Factor [CRF] Messenger Ribonucleic Acid [mRNA] and CRF-41 Peptide and Adenohypophysial Proopiomelanocortin mRNA During Chronic Inflammatory Stress. Endocrinology 1992; 130(3):1394-1400.

11. Patchev VK, Kalogeras KT, Zelazowski P, Wilder RL, Chrousos GP: Increased Plasma Concentrations, Hypothalamic Content, and in Vitro Release of Arginine Vasopressin in Inflammatory Disease-Prone, Hypothalamic Corticotropin Hormone-Deficient Lewis Rats. Endocrinology 1992; 131(3):1453-1457.

12. Swain MG, Patchev V, Vergalia J, Chrousos G, Anthony-Jones E: Suppression of Hypothalamic-Pituitary-Adrenal Axis Responsiveness to Stress in a Rat Model of Acute Cholestasis. J Clin Invest 1993; 91:1903-1908.

Sleep, Wakefulness, Neuroendocrine and Immune Function in Fibromyalgia and Chronic Fatigue Syndrome

Harvey Moldofsky

Chronic fatigue, diffuse musculoskeletal pain, light, unrefreshing sleep and cognitive-emotional distress are common features of chronic fatigue syndrome [CFS] and fibromyalgia syndrome [FS]. A comparison of symptoms in both these conditions shows that more than 90% of patients complain of disturbed sleep (1). Our studies of sleep physiology and symptoms of patients with CFS and FS reveal similar disordered sleep, namely an alpha [7.5-11 Hz] rhythm physiologic arousal disturbance in the electroencephalogram [EEG] during nonrapid eye movement [NREM] sleep that accompanies increased nocturnal vigilance and the light unrefreshing sleep (2-5). Recent studies confirm the EEG arousal disturbances in patients with CFS (6-8). The alpha EEG sleep anomaly and symptoms have been experimentally reproduced by noise disruption of stage 4 or slow wave [deep] sleep [SWS] in healthy sedentary subjects, but not in physically-fit runners (9). Some patients with CFS and FS have been also shown to have such primary sleep disorders as periodic involuntary limb movements or sleep apnea (10-15). Disturbed sleep and consequent sleep deprivation results in fatigue, sleepiness, impaired intellectual functioning and negative mood (16). These behavioral features are common to patients

Harvey Moldofsky, MD, is affiliated with the University of Toronto Centre for Sleep and Chronobiology, Western Division, The Toronto Hospital, 399 Bathurst Street, Toronto, Canada M5T 2S8.

[Haworth co-indexing entry note]: "Sleep, Wakefulness, Neuroendocrine and Immune Function in Fibromyalgia and Chronic Fatigue Syndrome." Moldofsky, Harvey. Co-published simultaneously in the *Journal of Musculoskeletal Pain* (The Haworth Medical Press, an imprint of The Haworth Press, Inc.) Vol. 3, No. 2, 1995, pp. 75-79; and: *Fibromyalgia, Chronic Fatigue Syndrome, and Repetitive Strain Injury: Current Concepts in Diagnosis, Management, Disability, and Health Economics* (ed: Andrew Chalmers et al.) The Haworth Medical Press, an imprint of The Haworth Press, Inc., 1995, pp. 75-79. Multiple copies of this article/chapter may be purchased from The Haworth Document Delivery Center [1-800-3-HAWORTH; 9:00 a.m. - 5:00 p.m. (EST)].

© 1995 by The Haworth Press, Inc. All rights reserved.

with CFS and FS. Our group and others (17,18,6,1) have proposed that altered sleep physiology and its relationship to the waking daytime symptoms are core ingredients to the pathology of CFS and of FS.

We have theorized that the symptoms of unrefreshing sleep, fatigue, diffuse myalgia, and psychologic distress involve a disorder in the chronobiology of the immune and neuroendocrine and sleep-wake systems of the brain (17,19). The chronobiologic theoretical model for CFS and FS is based on recent animal and human studies that show that the coordination of aspects of the immune-neuroendocrine and temperature rhythms of the body are intimately tied to the sleep-wake, brain-behavioral system (20). There is considerable experimental evidence for a molecular basis for the bidirectional communication between the immune and neuroendocrine systems (21-23). Not only do aspects of the immune and neuroendocrine systems interact, but also these systems influence or are influenced by the sleeping-waking brain. A variety of immunologically active peptides, such as interleukin-l [IL-1] and neuroendocrines, e.g., growth hormone releasing factor have been shown to promote sleep in animals (24,25). Krueger and Obal propose that the diurnal sleep-wake rhythm is the result of oscillatory mechanisms that involve brain IL-l and the neurohormones of the hypothalamic-pituitary axis. Our diurnal cytokine and cellular immune, and neuroendocrine studies in humans are consistent with this theory. Plasma IL-l and IL-2 relate to the sleep-wake cycle with maximal plasma IL-l occurring during SWS sleep (12,26). The IL-l-sleep relationship has been confirmed (27,28). In normal young males and females aspects of the peripheral cellular immune and neuroendocrine functions vary with sleep and wakefulness (12,29,30,26). Pokeweed mitogen response, an index of B cell lymphocyte function, is increased during nocturnal sleep and is inversely related to plasma cortisol. Natural killer [NK] cell activity declines with sleep and reaches its lowest levels in SWS during overnight sleep and during a series of naps over the course of a day (26). In women, the timing of the SWS and decline of NK activity differ with measures of plasma progesterone during the menstrual cycle (31). Recently, we showed that the proportion of NK cells in peripheral monocytes reaches its lowest point during SWS (31). The diurnal pattern of these cytokine and cellular immune and endocrine functions are altered with forty hours nocturnal sleep deprivation (29).

In patients with CFS, no specific viral etiology has been determined (32). Alterations in both the immune system (33-37) and the neuroendocrine system (38,39) have been implicated in the pathogenesis of the disorder. However, no confirmed or consistent abnormalities in cytokine, immunoglobulins, immune complexes and complement, cellular immune cells or cellular functions have been reported (33,34,35,37). The difficulties in interpreting the conflicting results in NK cells (33,34,35,37) T cell subsets or cytokines (33,34,35,37) may be the result of the reliance on single blood samples of those cellular or cytokine functions that are shown to vary over the sleep-wake cycle, and the influence of disordered sleep-wake physiology in CFS. In light of the evidence for an impairment of the hypothalamic-pituitary-adrenal axis (38) and the suggestion of reduced growth hormone secretion in FS (40) there is the possibility that central nervous system control of neuroendocrine and immune functions may be altered over the sleep-wake cycle in patients with CFS and in fibromyalgia. Studies on the interrelationships of the sleep-wake system of the brain, neuroimmune and neuroendocrine systems, are expected to further our understanding of the pathogenic mechanisms involved in these two disorders.

REFERENCES

1. Goldenberg, DL: Fibromyalgia and its relation to chronic fatigue syndrome, viral illness and immune abnormalities. J Rheumatol, (Suppl. 19) 16:91-93, 1989.

2. Moldofsky H, Scarisbrick P, England R, Smythe HA: Musculoskeletal symptoms and NonREM sleep disturbance in patients with "fibrositis syndrome" and healthy subjects. Psychosom Med, 34:341-351, 1975.

3. Moldofsky H, Lue FA: The relationship of alpha and delta EEG frequencies to pain and mood in fibrositis treated with chlorpromazine and L-tryptophan. EEG Clin Neurophys, 50:7180, 1980.

4. Anch AM, Lue FA, MacLean AW, Moldofsky H: Sleep physiology and psychological aspects of fibrositis (fibromyalgia syndrome). Can J Psychol, 45:179-184, 1991.

5. Whelton CL, Salit I, Moldofsky H: Sleep, Epstein-Barr virus infection, musculoskeletal pain, and depressive symptoms in chronic fatigue syndrome. J Rheumatol, 19:939-943, 1992.

6. Morriss R, Sharpe M, Sharpley AL, Cowen PJ, Hawton K, Morris J: Abnormalities of sleep in patients with the chronic fatigue syndrome. BMJ, 306:1161-1163, 1993.

7. Drewes AM, Nielsen KD, Jennum P, Andreasen A: Alpha intrusion in fibromyalgia. (Personal Communication), submitted for publication.

8. Carette S, Oakson G, Guimont C, Steriade M: Sleep electroencephalography (EEG) and the clinical response to amitriptyline in patients with fibromyalgia. Arth & Rheumat, 36(Suppl. 9):S250, 1993.

9. Moldofsky H, Scarisbrick P: Induction of neurasthenic musculoskeletal pain syndrome by selective sleep stage deprivation. Psychosom Med, 38:35-44, 1976.

10. Moldofsky H, Tullis C, Lue FA, Quance G, Davidson J: Sleep-related myoclonus in rheumatic pain modulation disorder (fibrositis syndrome) and in excessive daytime somnolence. Psychosom Med, 46:145-151, 1984.

11. Hamm C, Derman S, Russell IJ: Sleep parameters in fibrositis/fibromyalgia syndrome. Arth & Rheumat, 32:S70, 1989.

12. Molony RR, MacPeek DM, Schiffman PL, et al.: Sleep, sleep apnea and the fibromyalgia syndrome. J Rheumatol, 13:797-800, 1986.

13. Lario BA, Teran J, Alonso JL, Alegre J, Arroyo I, Viejo JL: Lack of association between fibromyalgia and sleep apnoea syndrome. Ann Rheum Dis, 51:108-111, 1992.

14. Jennum P, Drewes AM, Andreasen A, Neilsen KD: Sleep and other symptoms in primary fibromyalgia and in healthy controls. J Rheumatol 20:1756-1759, 1993.

15. May KP, West SG, Baker MR, Everett DW: Sleep apnea in male patients with fibromyalgia syndrome. Am J Med, 94:505-508, 1993.

16. Horne J: The functions of sleep in humans and other mammals. Oxford University Press, Oxford, 1988.

17. Moldofsky H: The chronobiology theory of fibromyalgia. J Musculoske Pain, 1(3,4):49-59,1993.

18. Bennett RM: The origin of myopain: An integrated hypothesis of focal muscle changes and sleep disturbance in patients with the fibromyalgia syndrome. J Musculoske Pain, 1(3,4):95-112, 1993.

19. Moldofsky H: Fibromyalgia, sleep disorder and chronic fatigue syndrome. In Chronic Fatigue Syndrome. Wiley, Chichester (Ciba Foundation Symposium, 173), pp 262-279, 1993b.

20. Moldofsky H: Immune-neuroendocrine-thermal mechanisms and the sleep-wake system. Sleep Onset Mechanisms. Edited by RD Ogilvie and JR Harsh. American Psychological Association (in press, 1994)

21. Blalock JE: A molecular basis for the bidirectional communication between the immune and neuroendocrine systems. Physiol Rev, 69:132, 1989.

22. Dunn AJ: Psychoneuroimmunology for the psychoneuro-endocrinologist: a review of animal studies of nervous system–immune interactions. Psychoneuroendocrinol, 14:251-274, 1989.

23. Daruna JH, Morgan JE: Psychosocial effects on immune function: neuroendocrine pathways. Psychosomatics, 31:4-12, 1990.

24. Krueger JM: Somnogenic activity *of* immune response modifiers. TIPS, 11:122-126, 1990.

25. Krueger JM, Obal F: A neuronal group theory of sleep functions. J Sleep Res, 2:63-69, 1993.

26. Shahal B, Lue FA, Jiang CG, MacLean A, Moldofsky H: Circadian and sleep-wake related changes in immune functions. J Sleep Res 1(Suppl):210, 1992.

27. Covelli V, Massari F, Fallarca C, Munno I, Jirrilo F, Savastano S, Tommaselli A, Lombardi G: Interleukin-1 beta and beta endorphin circadian rhythms are inversely related in normal and stress altered sleep. Int J Neurosci, 63:299-305, 1992.

28. Gudewill S, Pollmacher T, Vedder H, et al: Nocturnal plasma levels of cytokines in healthy men. Europ Arch Psychiatry & Clin Neurosci, 141:53-56, 1992.

29. Moldofsky H: Effects of sleep deprivation on human immune functions. FASEB J, 3:1972-1977, 1989.

30. Moldofsky H, Lue F, Shahal B, Jiang CG, Gorczynski RM: Circadian immune functions and the menstrual cycle in healthy women. Sleep Res, 20A:552, 1991.

31. Moldofsky H, Lue FA, Shahal B, Jiang CG, Gorczynski RM: Diurnal sleep/wake-related immune functions during the menstrual cycle of healthy young women. (Submitted, 1994).

32. Khan AS, Heneine WM, Chapman LE, Gary Jr HE, Woods TC, Folks TM, Schonberger LB: Assessment *of* a retrovirus sequence and other possible risk factors for the chronic fatigue syndrome in adults. Ann Intern Med, 118:241-245, 1993.

33. Buchwald D, Komaroff AI: Review of laboratory findings for patients with chronic fatigue syndrome. Rev Infectious Dis, 13(Suppl 1):S12S18, 1991.

34. Chao CC, Janoff EN, Hu S, Thomas K, Gallagher M, Tsang M, Peterson PK: Altered cytokine release in peripheral blood mononuclear cell cultures from patients with the chronic fatigue syndrome. Cytokine, 3:292-298, 1991.

35. Landay AL, Jessop C, Lennette ET, Levy JA: Chronic fatigue syndrome: clinical condition associated with immune activation. Lancet, 338[8769]:707-712, 1991.

36. Lloyd A, Hickie I, Hickie C, Dwyer J, Wakefield D: Cell mediated immunity in patients with chronic fatigue syndrome, healthy control subjects and patients with major depression. Clin Exp Immunol, 87:76-79, 1992.

37. Straus SE, Fritz S, Dale JK, Gould B, Strober W: Lymphocyte phenotype and function in the chronic fatigue syndrome. J Clin Immunol, 13:30-40, 1993.

38. Demitrack MA, Dale JK, Straus SE, Laue L, Listwak SJ, Kruesi MJP, Chrousos GP, Gold PW: Evidence for impaired activation of the hypothalamic pituitary adrenal axis in patients with chronic fatigue syndrome. J Clin Endocrinol Metab, 73:1224-1234, 1991.

39. Sternberg EM: Hyperimmune fatigue syndrome: diseases of the stress response. J Rheumatol, 20:418-421, 1993.

40. Bennett RM, Clark SR, Campbell SM, Buckhardt CS: Low levels of somatomedin C in patients with the fibromyalgia syndrome: a possible link between sleep and muscle pain. Arth & Rheumat, 35:1113-1116, 1992.

Comparing Fibromyalgia, Myofascial Pain, and Control Groups: A Search for Reliable Criteria

Eldon Tunks

SUMMARY. Despite differing clinical definitions, studies of fibromyalgia and myofascial pain have demonstrated common features, but few with adequate reliability to distinguish these conditions.

Empirical studies have been able to demonstrate reliable diagnostic criteria for diagnosis of fibromyalgia (1-4). In a multicenter study of chronic fibromyalgia and control subjects, conducted by fibromyalgia experts, a consensus was reached on diagnostic criteria for fibromyalgia (4). These criteria were diffuse pain reported on both sides and upper and lower body, trunk and limbs, and pain reported on palpation of 11 or more of 18 specified points. In comparing these criteria with those reached in other research papers, the differences are mainly in the number and choice of tender point locations, the degree of tenderness expected, and whether or not historical [anamnestic] symptoms were needed in the diagnosis.

The work of Kellgren in Lewis's laboratory provided an empirical basis for the study of referred pain (5,6) These findings and other clinical observations have since been organized into a clinical approach to muscle pain (7). Although numerous clinical studies have been carried out on myofascial pain, these for the most part do not address the reliability issues in diagnosis of myofascial pain.

Eldon Tunks, MD, FRCP[C], is Professor of Psychiatry, McMaster University, Chedoke-McMaster Hospital, Box 2000, Hamilton, Ontario, Canada L8N 3Z5.

[Haworth co-indexing entry note]: "Comparing Fibromyalgia, Myofascial Pain, and Control Groups: A Search for Reliable Criteria." Tunks, Eldon. Co-published simultaneously in the *Journal of Musculoskeletal Pain* (The Haworth Medical Press, an imprint of The Haworth Press, Inc.) Vol. 3, No. 2, 1995, pp. 81-85; and: *Fibromyalgia, Chronic Fatigue Syndrome, and Repetitive Strain Injury: Current Concepts in Diagnosis, Management, Disability, and Health Economics* (ed: Andrew Chalmers et al.) The Haworth Medical Press, an imprint of The Haworth Press, Inc., 1995, pp. 81-85. Multiple copies of this article/chapter may be purchased from The Haworth Document Delivery Center [1-800-3-HA-WORTH; 9:00 a.m. - 5:00 p.m. (EST)].

© 1995 by The Haworth Press, Inc. All rights reserved.

Several studies have cast some doubt on the clinical reliability of some key criteria of myofascial pain (8-10). There are clinical features that are commonly found in patients with myofascial pain and fibromyalgia. These include soft tissue pain at characteristic sites, regional or diffuse pain, and associated symptoms such as sleep disturbance and fatigue. In clinical practice, many cases are found of individuals who have features that are consistent with both fibromyalgia and myofascial pain criteria. One needs to know the reliability with which myofascial pain and fibromyalgia may be distinguished clinically from each other. A few empirical studies have compared fibromyalgia and myofascial subjects.

Scudds et al. (11), comparing a group of 20 fibromyalgia patients with 19 myofascial pain patients, found that fibromyalgia subjects had significantly greater pain responsiveness during dolorimetry, higher reported pain levels, lower general pain thresholds, and they reported pain diffusely whereas in the myofascial group, pain was likely to be reported in one body quadrant. Sleep was impaired similarly in these groups. Regional pain levels correlated with dolorimetry scores.

Durette et al. (12), comparing 21 myofascial patients with 4 with fibromyalgia, noted that tender points and trigger points were found in similar proportions in both the myofascial and fibromyalgia subjects.

Yunus, Masi, and Aldag (3) compared 63 fibromyalgia patients, 30 normal controls, 32 with rheumatoid arthritis, and 31 with traumatic fibromyalgia [localized musculoskeletal pain due to trauma or repetitive use]. The "traumatic fibromyalgia" group reported few of the characteristic historical features of fibromyalgia. The fibromyalgia and traumatic fibromyalgia groups differed on several subjective symptoms including "hurt all over," pain at 7 or more sites, general fatigue, poor sleep, anxiety and tension, and irritable bowel symptoms. Several tender point sites discriminated the traumatic from the fibromyalgia groups. The mean number of tender points in fibromyalgics was 5.9, contrasting with 1.1 among the traumatic fibromyalgics and 0.3 among normal controls. Criteria involving presence of tender points and anamnestic criteria were derived, which had 92% sensitivity and 94% specificity in discriminating fibromyalgia from either traumatic fibromyalgia or rheumatoid arthritis.

Jacobsen and Danneskiold-Samsoe (13) compared 36 patients with fibromyalgia and 18 with chronic myofascial pain. During a repetitive knee extension exercise, the myofascial pain subjects had a significantly greater dynamic muscular endurance with a more gradual decline in power than the fibromyalgia subjects.

A group of experts on myofascial pain and on fibromyalgia conducted blind clinical examinations on 23 women; 7 with fibromyalgia, 8 with myofascial pain, and 8 normal volunteers (10). The main point of the study was to establish the reliability with which key diagnostic features essential to the diagnoses of these conditions could be discriminated. The fibromyalgia experts found slightly more "tender points" in fibromyalgia patients than in myofascial patients. These groups did not differ with respect to taut bands, reproduction of the patients' clinical pain complaint by palpation, or tender points associated with referred pain or paresthesia, and there was poor reliability between fibromyalgia experts for the above findings. The myofascial experts found taut bands and twitches in all three subject groups. Fibromyalgia and myofascial subjects did not differ in regards to trigger point count, referred pain, nor in reproduction of the clinical pain problem by palpation. There was poor interobserver agreement on trigger point count, taut bands, and twitches. When minimal criteria [a very tender point with radiated pain] for "trigger points" were used, trigger points were found in 38% of fibromyalgia subjects and in 23% of myofascial subjects, but in less than 2% of normals.

Some studies have taken as an operational definition of myofascial pain the presence of tender points found in typical muscle regions and associated with referred or radiated pain (12). However, this may not be a stringent enough criterion for myofascial pain, since tender points with referred or radiated pain or paresthesia have also been found in fibromyalgia (2,12,14,15). Similarly, tender points and trigger points have been found together in both myofascial and fibromyalgia subjects (10,12).

The myofascial pain literature generally takes the position that trigger points [tender points that refer pain] are exquisitely tender (7). Orhbach and Gale (9) confirmed that the pain thresholds were lower for the points that referred pain, versus the points that produced local pain only.

Reproduction of clinical pain complaint by palpation of tender points is usually taken as a "major criterion" for myofascial pain, but pain reproduction by tender point stimulation has been reported also in fibromyalgia subjects (10). In a study of myofascial pain-dysfunction [affecting the temporomandibular joint system], referred pain had a poor correspondence to reported pain pattern and physical findings (9). Therefore, the relationship of referred pain to the reproduction of clinical pain complaint warrants further study.

While it is generally accepted that the diagnosis of myofascial pain currently relies on finding very tender areas with associated referred pain, the reliability of the diagnosis would depend on the reliability in clinical identification of these tender or trigger points. Poor reliability has been demonstrated in identification of bands and nodules (9,10), referred pain (9,16), reproduction of clinical pain by referred pain (9,10,16), and identification of trigger points (10,16). There is also some experimental evidence that significant inter- and intra-observer variation exists in identifying tender points (3).

In an empirical study of fibromyalgia, myofascial, pain controls who had neither myofascial nor fibromyalgia pain, and normal controls, blind raters demonstrated good inter-rater and test-retest reliability for dolorimetry and palpation-induced pain in tenderness assessment over 27 paired "tender point" and "control point areas" (16). The greatest tenderness by dolorimetry, and highest tender point counts, were found almost equally in the fibromyalgia and myofascial patients, with significantly fewer in the pain controls, and in the normals. However, these tender point counts and dolorimetry correlated weakly with location of patients' usual pain complaints. The frequency of referred pains correlated only with the number of tender points, regardless of the diagnosis.

REFERENCES

1. Yunus MB, Masi AT, Calabro JJ, Miller KA, Feigenbaum SL: Primary fibromyalgia [fibrositis]; clinical study of 50 patients with matched normal controls. Sem Arthritis Rheum 11: 151-171, 1981.

2. Campbell SM, Clark S, Tindall EA, Forehand ME, Bennett RM: Clinical characteristics of fibrositis; I. A "blinded" controlled study of symptoms and tender points. Arthritis Rheum 26: 817-824, 1983.

3. Yunus MB, Masi AT, Aldag JC: Preliminary criteria for primary fibromyalgia syndrome [PFS]; multivariate analysis of a consecutive series of PFS, other pain patients, and normal subjects. Clin Exp Rheumatol 7: 63-69, 1989.

4. Wolfe F, Smythe HA, Yunus MB, et al: The American College of Rheumatology 1990 criteria for the classification of fibromyalgia; Report of the Multicenter Criteria Committee. Arthritis Rheum 33: 160-172, 1990.

5. Kellgren JH: Observations on referred pain arising from muscle. Clin Sci 3: 175-190, 1938.

6. Kellgren JH: On the distribution of pain arising from deep somatic structures with charts on segmental pain areas. Clin Sci 4: 35-46, 1939.

7. Travell JG, Simons DG: Myofascial Pain and Dysfunction; The Trigger Point Manual. Williams and Wilkins, Baltimore, 1983, pp. 24-26.

8. Nice DA, Riddle DL, Lamb RL, Mayhew TP, Rucker K: Intertester reliability of judgments of the presence of trigger points with low back pain. Arch Phys Med Rehabil 73: 893-898. 1992.

9. Ohrbach R, Gale EN: Pressure pain thresholds, clinical assessment, and differential diagnosis; reliability and validity in patients with myogenic pain. Pain 39: 157-169, 1989.

10. Wolfe F, Simons DG, Fricton J, et al: The fibromyalgia and myofascial pain syndromes; a preliminary study of tender points and trigger points in persons

with fibromyalgia, myofascial pain syndrome, and no disease. J Rheumatol 19: 944-951, 1992.

11. Scudds RA, Trachsel LC, Luckhurst BJ, Percy JS: A comparative study of pain, sleep quality and pain responsiveness in fibrositis and myofascial pain syndrome. J Rheumatol 19 (Suppl): 120-126, 1989.

12. Durette MR, Rodriquez AA, Agre JC, Silverman JL: Needle electromyographic evaluation of patients with myofascial or fibromyalgic pain. Am J Phys Med Rehabil 70: 154-156, 1991.

13. Jacobsen S, Danneskiold-Samsoe B: Dynamic muscular endurance in primary fibromyalgia compared with chronic myofascial pain syndrome. Arch Phys Med Rehabil 73: 170-173, 1992.

14. Bengtsson A, Henriksson KG, Jorfeldt L, Kagedal B, Lennmarken C, Lindstrom F: Primary fibromyalgia; a clinical and laboratory study of 55 patients. Scand J Rheumatol 15: 340-347, 1986.

15. Simms, RW, Goldenberg DL: Symptoms mimicking neurological disorders in fibromyalgia syndrome. J Rheumatol 15: 1271-1273, 1988.

16. Tunks E, McCain GA, Hart LE, Teasell RW, Rollman GB, DeShane PJ, McDermid AJ, Goldsmith CH: The reliability of physical findings in patients with fibromyalgia and myofascial pain syndromes (abstract). Arthr Rheum (suppl.) 34: S190, 1991

Overlap of Fibromyalgia, Myofascial Pain, and Chronic Fatigue Syndrome

Don L. Goldenberg

SUMMARY. Objectives: To review common features seen in fibromyalgia, myofascial pain and chronic fatigue syndrome.

Methods: Informed literature review.

Results: Important common features are seen in these apparent disparate syndromes.

Conclusion: The striking similarity between these syndromes provides insight into potential pathogenetic and treatment options.

Fibromyalgia, myofascial pain, and chronic fatigue syndrome [CFS] are each termed syndromes. In contrast to a disease, these disorders have no known etiology or generally accepted pathology. In common with other syndromes, such as migraine and irritable bowel syndrome, physical and laboratory findings are not significantly abnormal or provide any diagnostic utility. However, syndromes are appropriate terms in order to describe homogeneous disorders that share common clinical features. Thus, the diagnosis of these disorders is based on symptoms and evolution of these symptoms over time. A consensus of experts have suggested classification criteria for both fibromyalgia and CFS (1,2). Formal classification criteria for myofascial pain have not been established (3). The diagnostic classifi-

---

Don L. Goldenberg, MD, is Chief of Rheumatology, Newton-Wellesley Hospital and Professor of Medicine, Tufts University School of Medicine.

Address correspondence to: Don Goldenberg, MD, Newton-Wellesley Hospital, 2014 Washington Street, Newton, MA 02162.

[Haworth co-indexing entry note]: "Overlap of Fibromyalgia, Myofascial Pain, and Chronic Fatigue Syndrome." Goldenberg, Don L. Co-published simultaneously in the *Journal of Musculoskeletal Pain* (The Haworth Medical Press, an imprint of The Haworth Press, Inc.) Vol. 3, No. 2, 1995, pp. 87-91; and: *Fibromyalgia, Chronic Fatigue Syndrome, and Repetitive Strain Injury: Current Concepts in Diagnosis, Management, Disability, and Health Economics* (ed: Andrew Chalmers et al.) The Haworth Medical Press, an imprint of The Haworth Press, Inc., 1995, pp. 87-91. Multiple copies of this article/chapter may be purchased from The Haworth Document Delivery Center [1-800-3-HAWORTH; 9:00 a.m. - 5:00 p.m. (EST)].

© 1995 by The Haworth Press, Inc. All rights reserved.

87

cation criteria for fibromyalgia were field-tested in a number of studies, with the most extensive completed in 1990 by the members of the American College of Rheumatology (1). Utilizing the simple classification criteria of widespread musculoskeletal pain and the presence of at least 11 of 18 possible tender points, fibromyalgia can be distinguished from other chronic rheumatic pain disorders with a high degree of specificity and sensitivity.

The classification criteria for myofascial pain has varied from one author to the next and there are no widely agreed upon criteria that have been tested. Myofascial pain is said to differ from fibromyalgia because the pain is regional and the characteristic physical finding is the trigger point, rather than the tender point. However, many patients may initially present with a regional pain syndrome which spreads to become a more generalized pain typical of fibromyalgia (3). Furthermore, the reliability and validity of the trigger point has been questioned. Trigger points, as tender points, are excessively tender on palpation, but also are characterized by a specific referral pattern of pain, and are found in a taut band of muscle which produces a twitch response when the muscle is lightly snapped (3). However, when experts in the diagnosis of fibromyalgia and in the diagnosis of myofascial pain examined patients with each condition, there was significant overlap in symptoms and tender points in both groups of patients. There was poor inter- and intra-rater reliability in the finding of trigger points and utilizing the above definition of a trigger point, the trigger point was uncommonly present in the muscle of patients with either fibromyalgia or myofascial pain syndrome (3). Patients with myofascial pain have similar sleep disturbances, fatigue and mood disturbances as reported in fibromyalgia. It has also been suggested that patients with myofascial pain respond better to focal therapy and generally have a self-limited pain condition, although controlled longitudinal trials or outcome studies have not been completed.

There is also a striking overlap of fibromyalgia and CFS. Both conditions have no known cause or well-documented pathologic abnormalities, both are more common in women, and both have similar symptoms, including severe fatigue, generalized myalgias, sleep disturbances, and neurocognitive and psychiatric symptoms (4). The initial Center for Disease Control [CDC] working case definition for CFS was recently revised to include the musculoskeletal features typical of fibromyalgia (5). Using operational classification criteria, we found that 70% of patients with fibromyalgia met the CDC definition of CFS (6). We also examined 30 randomly selected patients with CFS and found that two-thirds met the ACR classification criteria for fibromyalgia (7). Those CFS patients who had chronic myalgias each had at least 11 of the 18 positive tender points, whereas those CFS patients who did not complain of chronic myalgias had a normal tender point examination.

The descriptive history of fibromyalgia and CFS over the past century have many similarities (8). Of greatest interest has been a similar search for a causative agent, in particular an infection in the case of CFS, and for primary muscle pathology in fibromyalgia. Despite some initial evidence that the EBV virus or other putative viral agents are important in CFS, there is currently a consensus of opinion that no single infectious agent has been linked to this syndrome (5). However, there is strong clinical and some serologic evidence that various infectious agents may trigger or reactivate the symptoms of CFS in certain situations. There is also evidence that various infections, such as Lyme disease, may trigger or activate both fibromyalgia and CFS (9). Evidence for a primary pathologic process of muscle in fibromyalgia and CFS have followed similar pathways and have been unproductive. Although both conditions demonstrate similar non-specific structural, electromyographic, and biochemical changes, when appropriate sedentary controlled patients are compared, there are no significant differences regarding such changes (10,11).

Research in fibromyalgia and CFS recently has focused more on the central nervous system. There is a high prevalence of mood disturbances, particularly depression, in both conditions (12). Although this could simply be a reactive depression, family studies and lifetime history studies suggest that depression may be a biopsychologic marker of predisposition to these disorders. Similar sleep disturbances have been reported in fibromyalgia and CFS (13). Cognitive disturbances are well-documented in both conditions. Minor alterations of immune status, such as low NK cell activity, have been reported in both conditions (14). Current neurohormonal research has been directed at explaining these central nervous system findings with a unified hypothesis. Thus, abnormal serotonin metabolism (15), growth hormone activity (16), and hypothalamic-pituitary-adrenal axis dysfunction (17) provide further evidence for central mechanisms playing important roles in fibromyalgia and CFS.

In conclusion, there are striking similarities in these three syndromes. In understanding their pathogenesis, it seems logical to approach them similarly. A number of stressors, including infection, as well as physical and emotional trauma, may trigger a cascade of biopsychosocial changes that will include altered pain perception at central and peripheral levels, fatigue, mood disturbances, and sleep disturbances. Treatment in each of these syndromes should be directed to maladaptive psychosocial attitudes, especially those that foster inactivity, avoidance behavior, fear of infection and contagion, depression and feelings of helplessness and hopelessness.

REFERENCES

1. Wolfe F, Smythe HA, Yunus MB, et al: The American College of Rheumatology 1990 criteria for the classification of fibromyalgia: Report of the Multicenter Criteria Committee. Arthritis Rheum 33: 160-172, 1990.

2. Holmes GP, Kaplan JE, Gantz NM, et al: Chronic fatigue syndrome: a working case definition. Ann Intern Med 108: 387-389, 1988.

3. Wolfe F, Simons DG, Fricton J, et al: The fibromyalgia and myofascial pain syndromes: a preliminary study of tender points and trigger points in persons with fibromyalgia, myofascial pain syndrome and no disease. J Rheumatol 19: 944-951, 1992.

4. Goldenberg DL: Fibromyalgia and its relation to chronic fatigue syndrome, viral illness and immune abnormalities. J Rheumatol 16 (Suppl. 19): 91-93, 1989.

5. Schluederberg A, Straus SE, Peterson P, et al: Chronic fatigue syndrome research. Definition and medical outcome assessment. Ann Intern Med 117: 325-331, 1992.

6. Buchwald D, Goldenberg DL, Sullivan JL and Komaroff AL: The chronic, active Epstein-Barr virus infection: syndrome and primary fibromyalgia. Arthritis Rheum 30: 1132-1136, 1987.

7. Goldenberg DL, Simms RW, Geiger A and Komaroff AL: High frequency of fibromyalgia in patients with chronic fatigue seen in a primary care practice. Arthritis Rheum 33: 381-387, 1990.

8. Goldenberg DL: Fibromyalgia and other chronic fatigue syndromes: is there evidence for chronic viral illness? Semin Arthritis Rheum 18: 111-120, 1988.

9. Steere AC, Taylor E, McHugh GL and Logigian EL: The overdiagnosis of lyme disease. JAMA 269: 1812-1816, 1993.

10. Yunus MB and Kalyan-Raman UP: Muscle biopsy findings in primary fibromyalgia and other forms of nonarticular rheumatism. Rheum Dis Clin N Am 15: 115-134, 1989.

11. Lloyd AR, Gandevia SC and Hales JP: Muscle performance, voluntary activation, twitch properties and perceived effort in normal subjects and patients with the chronic fatigue syndrome. Brain 114: 85-98, 1991.

12. Hudson JI, Goldenberg DL, Pope HG,Jr., Keck PE,Jr. and Schlesinger L: Comorbidity of fibromyalgia with medical and psychiatric disorders. Am J Med 92: 363-367, 1992.

13. Whelton CL, Salit I, Moldofsky H: Sleep, Epstein-Barr virus infection, musculoskeletal pain, and depressive symptoms in chronic fatigue syndrome. J Rheumatol 19: 939-43, 1992.

14. Komaroff AL, Buchwald D: Symptoms and signs of chronic fatigue syndrome. Rev Infect Dis 13: S8-S11, 1991.

15. Russell IJ, Vaerqy H, Javors M, Nyberg F: Cerebrospinal fluid biogenic amine metabolites in fibromyalgia/fibrositis syndrome and rheumatoid arthritis. Arthritis Rheum 35: 550-556, 1992.

16. Bennett RM, Clark SR, Campbell SM and Burckhardt CS: Somatomedin-C levels in patients with the fibromyalgia syndrome: a possible link between sleep and muscle pain. Arthritis Rheum 35: 1113-1116, 1992.

17. Demitrack MA, Dale JK, Straus SE, et al: Evidence for impaired activation of the hypothalamic-pituitary-adrenal axis in patients with chronic fatigue syndrome. J Clin Endocrinol Metab 73: 1224-1234, 1991.

Is Myofascial Face Pain
a Regional Expression of Fibromyalgia?

Joseph J. Marbach

The diagnosis and treatment of myofascial face pain syndrome [MFP] has much in common with that of fibromyalgia syndrome [FS]. It may be merely an historical accident that separated how MFP and FS are viewed. In 1934 Costen, an otolaryngologist, described a syndrome that came to be called TMJ (1). Costen attributed the etiology of the facial pain to the loss of back teeth, not an uncommon state in the midst of the "great depression." For patients who had no missing teeth to replace, a bad bite or malocclusion was thought to cause the syndrome. Later, tooth grinding was added to the list of risk-factors. Control groups would have demonstrated that many people have missing teeth, malocclusions, and grind their teeth at night but do not suffer from face pain, and vice versa. Nevertheless, the relationship between MFP and dental etiologies remains strong. Like FS, MFP is known by a variety of names, e.g., TMJ, and myofascial type temporomandibular disorder [M/TMD].

The purpose of this paper is to examine the view that a special relationship exists between MFP and oral structures, thus separating MFP from FS. In the late 1940s, Schwartz (2) began a series of investigations. Instead of the usual meticulous examination of teeth, he introduced the meticulous examination of the patient. This approach has pointed in entirely new directions, by emphasizing the importance of epidemiology. Those who

Joseph J. Marbach, DDS, is Clinical Professor of Public Health, [Sociomedical Sciences] [in Psychiatry], School of Public Health and Department of Psychiatry, Columbia University, 600 West 168th Street, New York, NY 10032.

[Haworth co-indexing entry note]: "Is Myofascial Face Pain a Regional Expression of Fibromyalgia?" Marbach, Joseph J. Co-published simultaneously in the *Journal of Musculoskeletal Pain* (The Haworth Medical Press, an imprint of The Haworth Press, Inc.) Vol. 3, No. 2, 1995, pp. 93-97; and: *Fibromyalgia, Chronic Fatigue Syndrome, and Repetitive Strain Injury: Current Concepts in Diagnosis, Management, Disability, and Health Economics* (ed: Andrew Chalmers et al.) The Haworth Medical Press, an imprint of The Haworth Press, Inc., 1995, pp. 93-97. Multiple copies of this article/chapter may be purchased from The Haworth Document Delivery Center [1-800-3-HAWORTH; 9:00 a.m. - 5:00 p.m. (EST)].

© 1995 by The Haworth Press, Inc. All rights reserved.

sought care, for example, were mostly women [> 90%], mean age about 40 years, who reported many physical disorders besides MFP, appeared to be abnormally stressed psychologically, but whose teeth and bites showed no case/control differences. Schwartz was the first dentist to apply the treatment methods advocated by Travell to facial pain of muscle origin.

There are both short and long answers to the question posed in the title. If one applies the criteria established in 1990 by Wolfe et al. (3) the answer is no. FS is characterized by widespread or generalized aching and tenderness; myofascial syndromes are defined as regional. The longer answer requires examination of the 1990 criteria themselves. Note that 6 of 18 tender point sites [occiput, low cervical, and trapezius] are also MFP sites. Historical factors mentioned above prevented the masseter, temporalis, digastric, the body of the sternocleidomastoid and perhaps the internal and external pterygoid muscles from inclusion in the FS tender point list. Were these muscles to be given equal status with the other 12 non-overlapping tender point sites a more anatomically comprehensive picture of FS would emerge. Furthermore, risk-factors for, and patient characteristics of, FS and MFP overlap. The chief separation are aspects specifically associated with dental factors.

There is no satisfactory explanation for the consistently high ratio of females [> 90%] to males who seek care for MFP. Epidemiologic data report, however, that the symptoms of MFP exist only about twice as often among females (4). These studies attempt to distinguish between rates of subjects from whom isolated signs and symptoms are elicited and rates of MFP itself. The rates of isolated signs and symptoms are probably distributed quite differently from the actual rates of MFP. The likelihood that MFP is, as FS, more prevalent in women suggests that special attention be paid to distinctively female health and social issues.

When compared to controls, more ever-married MFP cases are childless. This is so, despite on average, that they were similar with respect to marital status, age, sexual activity, and contraceptive use. With respect to premenstrual pain, cases report significantly more headaches, back, joint or muscle pains, and abdominal pains than do controls (5). Indeed when compared to controls, cases are also beleaguered by physical illnesses and injuries as well as the pain associated with MFP. Table 1 compares demographic and physical variables of MFP cases and their controls with FS cases.

It is widely accepted that abnormal personality traits are important factors in the etiology and maintenance of the MFP. However, the foundation of this belief rests largely on clinical lore rather than evidence. Contrary to uncontrolled earlier studies, there appears to exist few personality characteristics (6) that distinguish MFP cases from properly selected controls.

TABLE 1. Pain Complaints and Symptoms for Myofascial Face Pain,[1,2] Their Non-MFP Controls,[1,2] and Fibromyalgia Patients.[3]

Variable	MFP [N = 151-158]	MFP-CONTROL [N = 132-139]	FS[3] N = 158
Age in years, Mean [s.d.]	38.0 [11.7][1]	39.9 [11.5][1]	44.7 [10.41]
Sex [% female]	100[1,2]	100[1,2]	92.4
Ethnic group [% Caucasian]	100[1,2]	100[1,2]	91.1
Patient-rated severity			
Pain [0-100] scale			62.3 [25.0]
Current Pain	30.0 [21][1]		
Worst Pain of Month	57.0 [24][1]		
Sleep disturbance	57.0[1]		75.6
Fatigue	72.0[1]	28.8[1]	78.2
Migraines	39.0[2]	28.8[2]	
Tension headaches	40.5[2]	34.0[2]	
Headaches			54.3
Irritable bowel	50.6[2]	27.2[2]	35.7
Myofascial back pain	40.5[2]	15.1[2]	
Myofascial neck pain	46.2[2]	24.2[2]	
Back pain	34.2[2]	23.5[2]	
Fibromyalgia	23.4[2]	0.0[2]	

The Ns differ slightly because the MFP and their control data are derived from two different cohorts. MFP data designated [1] are from Marbach et al., 1988; MFP data designated [2] are from an ongoing incomplete study consisting of 158 cases and 132 controls. Because half the cases and controls selected had a life-time history of at least one episode of major depression as measured by a semi-structured psychiatric interview, these data cannot be considered representative of MFP cases or non-MFP controls, but are provided only as exploratory. For each disorder all findings are life-time, not necessarily current rates. The Ns will eventually be 160 for each group, so that these data are likely to change somewhat especially for the control group. The FS data [3] are from Wolfe et al., 1990. [4] Values are the percentage of patients who reported pain on manual palpation examination: masseter [82.1], sternocleido-mastoid [76.8], splenius capitis [68.9], temporalis [66.9], trapezius [58.9] (Raphael & Marbach, 1992) and from [2] occipital pain [23.4].

There are a variety of potential sources of bias and error in many studies of the psychology of chronic pain. For example, many cases who find their way into research projects are also those who are the most chronically ill. Beleaguered by repeated episodes of pain, it is not surprising that chronic cases experience increased emotional distress. Rather than the emotional state representing the causative factor, many studies find that the physiological, behavioral, and cognitive consequences of chronic pain form a feedback loop that exacerbates the pain. Furthermore, depression, social isolation and lack of physical activity often accompanies chronic pain. Thus far, our findings show stress as an exacerbator, not as a cause of pain.

Tooth grinding and its treatment with various oral devices have assumed a central place in the MFP lore. To study the role of tooth grinding in MFP, cases and controls were asked about current and past tooth grinding (5). Cases were not significantly more likely than controls to report that they tooth grind. They were, however, significantly more likely to report that a dentist had told them they grind. These findings are consistent with the proposition that self-reports of grinding may be influenced by the treating clinician. Clinicians should not recommend oral devices considering their high cost, and the recent finding that they were no better than placebo in reducing MFP pain (7). Indeed, oral devices like most objects [food, pens, chewing gum] that people place in their mouths stimulate chewing. Tooth marks observed on the devices have probably contributed to the belief that MFP cases grind at night, when it is the device that promotes the grinding.

DISCUSSION

Myofascial face pain and fibromyalgia share in common many features. Their demographic, physical, and psychological characteristics are similar. Recognition and further analysis may allow for new insights into chronic facial pain.

REFERENCES

1. Costen JB: A syndrome of ear and sinus symptoms dependent upon disturbed function of the temporomandibular joint. Ann Otolaryngol 43:1-15, 1934.

2. Schwartz L: Disorders of the Temporomandibular Joint. W.B. Saunders, Philadelphia, 1959.

3. Wolfe F, Smythe HA, Yunus MB, Bennett RM, Bombardier C, Goldenberg DL, Tugwell P, Campbell SM, Abeles M, Clark P, Fan AG, Farber SJ, Fiechtner JJ, Franklin CM, Gatter RA, Hamaty D, Lessard J, Lichtbroun AS, Masi AT,

McCain GA, Reynolds WJ, Romano TJ, Russell IJ, Sheon RP: The American College of Rheumatology 1990 Criteria for the Classification of Fibromyalgia. Arthritis and Rheumatism 33: 160-172, 1990.

4. Lipton JA, Ship JA, Larch-Robinson D: Estimated prevalence and distribution of reported orofacial pain in the United States. JADA 124:115-121, 1993.

5. Marbach JJ, Lennon MC, Dohrenwend BP: Candidate risk factors for temporomandibular pain and dysfunction syndrome: psychosocial, health behavior, physical illness and injury. Pain 34: 139-151, 1988.

6. Marbach JJ: The "temporomandibular pain dysfunction syndrome" personality: fact or fiction? Journal of Oral Rehabilitation 19: 545-560, 1992.

7. Dao TTT, Lavigne GJ, Charbonneau A, Feine JS, Lund JP: The efficacy of oral splints in the treatment of myofascial pain of the jaw muscles: a controlled clinical trial. Pain 56: 85-94, 1994.

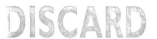
DISCARD

The Role of Joint Dysfunction in Spinal Myofascial Pain

Howard Vernon

SUMMARY. Objective: To review evidence relating to spinal mechanisms and peripheral pain and tenderness.

Findings and conclusions: Abnormalities of spinal function may associate with clinical features deemed characteristic of myofascial pain syndromes and fibromyalgia: Attention to such mechanisms may provide a unifying hypothesis for apparently different clinical phenomena.

INTRODUCTION

The aim of this presentation is to call greater attention amongst myofascial pain specialists to the role of spinal segmental dysfunction in regional [myofascial pain dysfunction [MPD]] and generalized fibromyalgia [FS] pain syndromes. We are challenged to do this because of a variety of clinical phenomena, including:

A. The existence of the classic "rheumatologic crux" which implies a high prevalence of cervical and lumbar-pelvic pain in myofascial pain patients (1);

B. Spinal tender or trigger points [TPs] are prominent components of MPD (2,3);

Howard Vernon, DC, FCCS, is Associate Dean, Canadian Memorial Chiropractic College, 1900 Bayview Avenue, Toronto, Ontario, Canada M4G 3E6.

[Haworth co-indexing entry note]: "The Role of Joint Dysfunction in Spinal Myofascial Pain." Vernon, Howard. Co-published simultaneously in the *Journal of Musculoskeletal Pain* (The Haworth Medical Press, an imprint of The Haworth Press, Inc.) Vol. 3, No. 2, 1995, pp. 99-104; and: *Fibromyalgia, Chronic Fatigue Syndrome, and Repetitive Strain Injury: Current Concepts in Diagnosis, Management, Disability, and Health Economics* (ed: Andrew Chalmers et al.) The Haworth Medical Press, an imprint of The Haworth Press, Inc., 1995, pp. 99-104. Multiple copies of this article/chapter may be purchased from The Haworth Document Delivery Center [1-800-3-HAWORTH; 9:00 a.m. - 5:00 p.m. (EST)].

© 1995 by The Haworth Press, Inc. All rights reserved.

    C. The high propensity for chronicity to develop in spinal pain syndromes (4);

    D. The high propensity for recurrence in spinal [myofascial] pain syndromes (4);

    E. The high propensity for spinal pain to be referred to distal sites, whereas the converse occurs much less frequently (4).

This last point may be the most important in pointing to a unique characteristic of spinal dysfunction in the development of myofascial pain.

Finally, the favorable results of clinical trials of spinal manipulation for low back, pelvic and neck pain syndromes as well as for headaches probably implicates myofascial pain as a target of spinal manipulation. Anecdotal evidence exists for relief of pain with spinal manipulation in MPD and FS (5).

DISCUSSION

What Is the Nature of Spinal Segmental Dysfunction?

Spinal segmental dysfunction is generally characterized by disturbance in alignment and/or motion characteristics of the vertebral motion segment, most especially a loss of motion or hypomobility. The notion of such articular dysfunction in the spine has been one of the cornerstones of the clinical models of chiropractic, osteopathy, manual medicine and manipulative physiotherapy. Mechanisms which have been proposed to explain spinal dysfunction include: intra-articular loss of joint play, intra-articular joint inclusions, sustained contraction or contracture of the deep segmental muscles, and disc fragmentation. Others have opted not to define or explicate this lesion, preferring, simply to call it "the manipulable lesion" (6).

As Lewit has pointed out (7), all of these explanatory models have as their basis the phenomenon of a barrier to joint motion. The "normal barrier" has a "soft end feel" with little sense of tension or pain. Dysfunction is characterized by a firmer barrier occurring earlier in the range of motion, increased tension, and pain. Sandoz speaks of a "paraphysiologic space" where, when a manipulation is performed, cavitation occurs, joint co-aptation is decreased and joint mobility is increased.

Lewit has further summarized other evidence for articular dysfunction in the spine, such as: "there are joints that are neither moved nor opposed by muscles, and yet can be restricted in movement" [sacroiliac, acromioclavicular, sterno clavicular, tibiofibular]; "joint play is most severely affected in movement [dysfunction], although it cannot be carried out by muscles and is only slightly opposed by them"; and joint [dysfunction] diagnosed prior to surgery can still be detected under general anesthesia with muscle relaxants. "This has spawned renewed interest in manipulation under anesthesia."

Are Spinal Joints Capable of Initiating Pain?

Nociceptor innervation of the spinal joints, ligaments and facet capsules has been amply demonstrated in the literature, most particularly by Giles (9,10). Posterior motion segment tissues receive their nociceptor innervation via a variety of pathways including: the lateral, intermediate and, especially [for articular tissues] medial branches of the posterior primary ramus, the recurrent meningeal nerve and other paravertebral nerves. Giles has utilized a number of sophisticated techniques to identify nociceptor innervation in lumbar joint capsules and synovial folds. These techniques include substance P immuno-histochemistry, silver and gold chloride impregnation and immuno-fluorescence studies.

Can the Spinal Joints Create Local and Referred Myofascial Pain and Tenderness?

Sinclair et al., Lewis, and Kellgren (11,12,13) published now-classic studies in the mid-century in which pain from the deep spinal ligaments [interspinous, facet joint capsules] in humans was provoked by the injection of algesic stimulants [i.e., hypertonic saline]. Pain from the spinal joints was typically felt both locally in the adjacent paraspinal regions as well as in remote or referred regions which appeared to be organized segmentally. Evidence with regard to the sacroiliac joint ligaments demonstrates widespread pain referral into the pelvic girdle and lower extremity. Feinstein's classic work (14) mapped these local and referred pain patterns from each facet level in normal human subjects. It is readily apparent that the typical pain patterns arising from facet joint irritation greatly resemble and could easily be mistaken for focal pain points which have been identified by others as the myofascial points typical of regional or widespread myofascial dysfunction.

What Is the Association Between Spinal Joint Dysfunction and Pain?

The association of spinal joint dysfunction and local or referred myofascial pain and tenderness has typically been explored by determining the level of concordance of separate and, hopefully, independent examinations for joint motion, on the one hand, and soft tissue pain/tenderness on the other.

Our group has undertaken two such studies, one involving thoracic spine dysfunction (15), and the other involving the lumbar region [unpublished data]. In both studies, independent, blinded examiners first determined the location of active paraspinal tender points, utilizing in the thoracic group, skin-rolling, and, in the lumbar group, scanning digital palpation. The next examiner measured the pressure pain threshold [PPT] with an algometer at the site of the tender points and at control points located contralaterally above or below the test level. A third examiner conducted prone motion palpation tests for intervertebral rotation and A-P glide between T4-T10 in the thoracic study and T12-L5 in the lumbar study. Only findings of major blockage were accepted as a positive test.

In the thoracic study, a large, statistically significant difference was found in PPT levels between tender points and control points. The Kappa value for concordance between tender points and major blockage within one segment above or below was 0.46, indicating a moderate level of association. In the lumbar spine a Kappa value of 0.67 was determined. As well, when the number of tender points was compared to the number of fixations, a highly significant Chi Square distribution was determined. It must be borne in mind that the cutaneous innervation of the paraspinal region derives from at least 3 spinal segments in the lumbar spine and up to 5 segments in the thoracic region. As such, these data can be interpreted to imply a mild to moderately high level of association in certain spine pain patients between paraspinal myofascial tenderness and subjacent motion segment hypomobility.

What Do Animal Studies Reveal About Spinal Dysfunction and Myofascial Pain?

Animal experimental studies of spinal joint pain are very few in number. Two groups have reported on experimental algesic studies. In 1993, Gillette et al. (16) reported on the results of algesic stimulation using bradykinin and hypertonic saline injected into a variety of deep segmental tissues including the multifidus muscles, facet joints, disc, and sympathetic ganglia. Using single unit extra-cellular recordings of dorsal horn neurons, they demonstrated that there is a remarkable diversity of sources of input to these cells, including from the posterior joint capsule, multifidus muscle, intervertebral disc, dura mater, sympathetic ganglia and peripheral musculature. This phenomenon was termed "hyperconvergence." These units had very large and often bilateral cutaneous receptive fields which extended well into the lower limbs. After algesic stimulation, very large expansions of the cutaneous and deep receptive fields of these neurons as well as higher levels of spontaneous firing occurred. These findings are consistent with the phenomenon of "central sensitization" reported by Woolf [see ref. 17] with the exception that the extent of increase or expansion of receptive fields induced by stimulation of axial [spinal] tissues appeared to be greater than that obtained by other researchers by stimulation of distal extremity tissues [i.e., hind limb musculature, knee joint. See below].

In 1993, Hu et al. (17) reported on excitatory effects in local and remote neck and jaw muscles of algesic stimulation in the deep para-articular structures of the upper cervical spine in the rat. These effects were elicited by injection of the C fiber irritant mustard oil and were compared to vehicle controls. Mustard oil evoked strong immediate EMG increases in local deep ipsilateral superficial neck muscles [rectus capitis posticus], local ipsilateral superficial neck muscles [trapezius] and remote ipsilateral jaw muscles [masseter and digastric] implying a divergent widespread activation pattern produced by experimental spinal pain. Additionally these increases in EMG were seen in two distinct phases–an early phase, lasting 3-4 minutes, and a late phase, occurring after a 10-minute suppression phase, and lasting for up to 20 minutes. In a subsequent study by Yu et al. involving mustard oil injected in the TMJ, only jaw muscles but not neck muscles demonstrated increases in EMG levels adding further support to the findings of Gillette et al. that algesic stimulation of axial/spinal structures may produce more profound facilitatory or sensitizing effects on somato-sensory and sensori-motor reflex mechanisms than does algesic stimulation of peripheral structures.

This, amongst other yet-to-be-determined mechanisms, may explain the much greater propensity for proximal and even more so, axial somatic structures to create referred pain projections in clinical disorders such as MPD and fibromyalgia.

REFERENCES

1. Cyriax J: Textbook of Orthopaedic Medicine. Vol.1. Diagnosis of Soft Tissue Lesions. London; Bailliere, Tindall and Cassell, 1969.

2. Travell JG and Simons DG: Myofascial Pain and Dysfunction: The Trigger Point Manual. Baltimore; Williams and Wilkens, 1983.

3. Travell J and Rinzler SH: Myofascial genesis of pain. Postgrad Med: 425-434, 1952.

4. Haldeman S: The neurophysiology of spinal pain syndromes. Edited by S Haldeman. Modern Developments in the Principles and Practice of Chiropractic. New York, Appleton-Century-Crofts, 1980.

5. Wolfe F: The clinical syndrome of fibrositis. Am J Med 81:81, 1986.

6. Haldeman S: Why one cause of back pain? Edited by AA Buerger and TS Tobis. Approaches to the Validation of Manipulative Therapy. Springfield, IL. Thomas, 1977.

7. Lewit K: Management of muscular pain associated with articular dysfunction. J Man Med 6:140-142, 1991.

8. Breen A: Integrated spinal motion: a study of two cases. J Can Chirop Assoc 35(1):25-30, 1991.

9. Giles LGF: The Anatomical Basis of Low Back Pain. Baltimore, MD. Williams and Wilkens, 1989.

10. Giles LGF and Harvey AR: Immunohistochemical demonstration of nociceptors in the capsule and synovial folds of human zygapophyseal joints. Br J Rheum 26:363-364, 1987.

11. Sinclair DC, Feindel WH, Weddell G, Falconer MA: The intervertebral ligaments as a source of segmental pain. J Bone Joint Surg 30B:515-521, 1948.

12. Lewis T: Experiments relating to cutaneous hyperalgesia and its spread through somatic fibers. Clin Sci 2:373-423, 1935.

13. Kellgren JH and Lewis T: Observations related to referred pain, visceromotor reflexes and other associated phenomena. Clin Sci 4:47, 1934.

14. Feinstein B: Referred pain from paravertebral structures. Edited by A A Buerger and JS Tobis. Approaches to the Validation of Manipulative Therapy. Springfield, IL. Thomas, 1978.

15. Taylor P, Tole G, Vernon HT: Skin rolling technique as an indicator of spinal joint dysfunction. J Can Chirop Assoc 34(2):82-86, 1990.

16. Gillette RG, Kramis RC, Roberts WJ: Characterization of spinal somatosensory neurons having receptive fields on lumbar tissues of cats. Pain 54(1):85-98, 1993.

17. Hu JW, Yu X-M, Vernon HT, Sessle BJ: Excitatory effects on neck and jaw muscle activity of inflammatory irritant applied to cervical paraspinal tissues. Pain 55:243-250, 1993.

Psychosocial Dysfunction
and Chronic Fatigue Syndrome

Susan E. Abbey

Chronic fatigue syndrome [CFS] is associated with significant psychosocial disability including marked impairment in the ability to function occupationally, socially and recreationally. Interpersonal relationships are strained by the unpredictability of the patient's functioning and the frequent need for others to assume a greater share of responsibilities, both instrumental and emotional, than in the past. This can result in lost friendships, strained marriages and disrupted family relationships. Finally, many CFS patients report the inability to pursue formerly pleasurable avocational activities which had been an important source of gratification, self-esteem and had been effective in reducing stress and modulating their emotional state.

Recent follow-up studies of CFS patient samples have emphasized the importance of psychological factors including psychiatric diagnosis, attitudes towards the illness, illness attributions and coping style in outcome (1,2,3). Wilson et al. (3) concluded that, "Psychological factors such as illness attitudes and coping style seem more important predictors of long-term outcome than immunological and demographic variables." The assessment of psychosocial dysfunction and treatment strategies related to the optimization of such functioning should be an integral part of the care of CFS patients. This paper will review the limited literature on psychoso-

Susan E. Abbey, MD, FRCP[C], is affiliated with the Department of Psychiatry, 8 EN-212, The Toronto Hospital, 200 Elizabeth Street, Toronto, Ontario, Canada M5G 2C4.

[Haworth co-indexing entry note]: "Psychosocial Dysfunction and Chronic Fatigue Syndrome." Abbey, Susan E. Co-published simultaneously in the *Journal of Musculoskeletal Pain* (The Haworth Medical Press, an imprint of The Haworth Press, Inc.) Vol. 3, No. 2, 1995, pp. 105-110; and: *Fibromyalgia, Chronic Fatigue Syndrome, and Repetitive Strain Injury: Current Concepts in Diagnosis, Management, Disability, and Health Economics* (ed: Andrew Chalmers et al.) The Haworth Medical Press, an imprint of The Haworth Press, Inc., 1995, pp. 105-110. Multiple copies of this article/chapter may be purchased from The Haworth Document Delivery Center [1-800-3-HAWORTH; 9:00 a.m. - 5:00 p.m. (EST)].

© 1995 by The Haworth Press, Inc. All rights reserved.

cial adjustment in CFS, ways of coping with the illness, and current perspectives on the necessary components of a psychosocial evaluation directed towards psychosocial rehabilitation and treatment of the patient with CFS.

PRECIPITATING, INITIATING AND MAINTAINING FACTORS IN CFS

While there is still much to be learned about the predisposing and precipitating or initiating factors with regards to CFS, there has been the increasing recognition that, as with many other medical diagnoses, the factors which are important in maintaining functional disability may be *different* from those which initiated it. Psychosocial factors and dysfunction may be important in maintaining or reinforcing poor functioning in the CFS long after the initiating events are no longer contributory. Wessely et al. (4) proposed that for many patients an initial infective trigger begins a cycle in which both attributional and cognitive factors trigger avoidant behavior and this in itself sustains symptoms. Similarly, depression and demoralization may sustain symptoms and may be triggered by attributional and cognitive factors, avoidance behavior or a variety of other pathophysiological mechanisms (4). This model of psychosocial perpetuating factors delineates treatment targets and emphasizes the necessity of addressing these factors in order for the CFS patient to reach optimal levels of functioning.

Evidence from the study of functional disorders such as irritable bowel syndrome has shown that there are differential levels of psychiatric morbidity, psychosocial distress and thus of the complexity of intervention required depending on where patients are seen. In general, patients seen in primary care settings have lower rates of psychiatric diagnoses and psychosocial distress and require less complex interventions than do those seen in tertiary care settings (5).

PSYCHIATRIC DISORDERS AND PSYCHOSOCIAL DYSFUNCTION

Psychiatric disorders are commonly diagnosed in patients with CFS (6), although there is considerable debate as to the meaning of these research findings (6,7). Nonetheless, what does seem to be clear, based on anecdotal reports from clinicians and supported by research observations (4), is that the effective treatment of mood and anxiety disorder diagnoses is essential prior to embarking on a rehabilitation program. In a pilot study of cognitive-behavioral therapy conducted by Wessely and colleagues, major depression was the most important predictor of failed response to treatment (4).

COPING STYLES AND ILLNESS

Coping refers to the cognitive and physical approaches used to achieve an optimal level of functioning including restoring reversibly impaired functions, compensating for irreversible impairments and maintaining some sense of bodily and psychic integrity. A variety of different coping strategies have been described but they can basically be divided into the two broad categories of engagement and disengagement from the stressful life situation. In general, disengaged or avoidant coping strategies are associated with poorer outcome. Questions remain as to the directionality of the relationship between coping strategies and outcome. The chronic pain literature has demonstrated that negative pain-related cognitions and passive pain-coping strategies have been associated with greater pain intensity, behavioral disruption, heightened distress, poor adjustment and negative affect (8). Avoidance sustains and augments psychosocial dysfunction in patients with chronic pain (8) and leads to a decreased sense of control, increased expectations that exposure will increase pain which in turn leads to further withdrawal from normal activities, and a decreased tolerance for activities (8).

COPING STRATEGIES IN CFS

There have been three studies of coping strategies in CFS (9,10,11) which found: increased use of avoidance (9); that maintaining activity was associated with higher functioning but more anxiety and that focusing on symptoms was associated with negative implications for impairment and emotional adjustment (10); and that more maladaptive cognitive appraisals and more frequent use of disengagement/denial coping strategies was associated with greater disturbances in both physical and psychosocial domains (11). A transactional model was proposed in which cognitive-behavioral processes operate to perpetuate the severity of other processes in a disordered system (11). Thus, exacerbation of symptoms evaluated by maladaptive appraisals and dealt with by less adaptive coping responses could result in the activation of affective, neuroendocrine and immunological pathways which would in turn further exacerbate symptoms (11).

IMPLICATIONS OF PRELIMINARY STUDIES
ON COPING AND CFS

These preliminary studies on coping and CFS support the potential efficacy of cognitive-behavioral interventions in increasing the functional occupational, social and recreational or avocational capacities of individuals with CFS. It is possible to use these strategies to modify maladaptive cognitive appraisals and to develop coping strategies which are associated with better outcomes in this group. Interventions are based upon a comprehensive psychosocial assessment of the CFS patient [see Table 1]. A careful delineation of these variables will direct the physician and treatment team in prioritizing treatment needs and sequencing appropriate treatments. The comprehensive assessment of patients with CFS typically

TABLE 1. The comprehensive assessment of psychosocial function in the patient with CFS.

1. PSYCHIATRIC DISORDERS

    Axis I Psychiatric Disorders
            major depression
            dysthymia
            panic disorder
            generalized anxiety disorder
            somatoform disorders
            substance use disorders
            sleep disorders

    Axis II Personality Disorders

2. PSYCHOSOCIAL STRESSORS

    current and past traumatic events
    interpersonal difficulties [marital, family, friends]
    work-related stressors

3. BELIEFS AND ATTRIBUTIONS REGARDING CFS

4. BEHAVIORAL PATTERNS

            behavioral avoidance
            bursts of activity

5. COPING STRATEGIES

yields more than one appropriate target for treatment. Treatment planning involves assigning priorities to these different issues and then devising the most cost-effective plan for intervening. Clinical experience with rehabilitation approaches to CFS suggest that it is essential to treat major depression, if it is present, prior to embarking on specific rehabilitation activities. While the treatment of CFS is beyond the scope of this article, it should be noted that a variety of treatment strategies have been proposed to ameliorate the psychosocial dysfunction associated with CFS (12,13).

CONCLUSIONS

Psychosocial dysfunction is a cause of significant distress and suffering for CFS patients and their families. While we have much yet to learn about the psychosocial rehabilitation of patients with CFS, initial studies in CFS and studies in other potentially related disorders suggest that psychosocial rehabilitation is possible and with it there is an improved quality of life.

REFERENCES

1. Sharpe M, Hawton K, Seagrott V, Pasvol G: Follow up of patients presenting with fatigue to an infectious diseases clinic. Br Med J 305:147-152, 1993.

2. Bonner D, Ron M, Chalder T, Butler S, Wessely S: Chronic fatigue syndrome: a follow up study. J Neurol Neurosurg Psychiatry 57:617-621, 1994.

3. Wilson A, Hickie I, Lloyd A, Hadzi-Pavlovi D, Boughton C, Dwyer J, Wakefield D: Longitudinal study of outcome of chronic fatigue syndrome. Br Med J 08:756-759, 1994.

4. Wessely S, Butler S, Chalder T, David A: The cognitive behavioral management of the post-viral fatigue syndrome: Post-Viral Fatigue Syndrome. Edited by R Jenkins, J Mowbray. John Wiley & Sons, Chichester, 1991, pp. 305-334.

5. Drossman DA, Thompson WG: Irritable bowel syndrome: review and a graduated multi-component treatment approach. Ann Intern Med 116:1009-1016, 1992.

6. Katon WJ, Walker EA: The relationship of chronic fatigue to psychiatric illness in community, primary care and tertiary care samples: Chronic Fatigue Syndrome (Ciba Foundation Symposium 173). Edited by GR Bock, J Whelan. Wiley, Chichester, 1993 pp. 193-211.

7. Abbey SE, Garfinkel PE: Chronic fatigue syndrome and depression: cause, effect, or covariate. Rev Inf Dis 13(Suppl 1):S73-83, 1991.

8. Sternbach RA (ed). The Psychology of Pain, Second Edition. New York: Raven Press, 1986.

9. Blakely AA, Howard RC, Sosich RM, Murdoch JC, Menkes DB, Spears GFS: Psychiatric symptoms, personality and ways of coping in chronic fatigue syndrome. Psychol Med 21:347-362, 1991.

10. Ray C, Weir W, Stewart D, Miller P, Hyde G: Ways of coping with chronic fatigue syndrome: development of an illness management questionnaire. Soc Sci Med 37:385-391, 1993.

11. Antoni MH, Brickman A, Lutgendorf S, Klimas N, Imia-Fins A, Ironson G, Quillian R, Miguez MJ, van Riel F, Morgan R, Patarca R, Fletcher MA: Psychosocial correlates of illness burden in chronic fatigue syndrome. Clin Infect Dis 18(Suppl 1):S73-78, 1994.

12. Sharpe M: Non-pharmacological approaches to treatment: Chronic Fatigue Syndrome, CIBA Foundation Symposium 173. Edited by GR Brock, J Whelan, John Wiley & Sons, Toronto, 1993, pp. 298-317.

13. Abbey SE: Psychopharmacology and chronic fatigue syndrome: Chronic Fatigue Syndrome. Edited by SE Straus, Marcel Dekker, New York, 1994 pp. 405-434.

Social and Cultural Aspects
of Chronic Fatigue Syndrome

Simon Wessely

Patients with chronic exhaustion after minimal effort for which a medical explanation is lacking are not new. In the past they have been labelled as suffering from neurasthenia, neurocirculatory asthenia, nervous exhaustion, effort syndrome and others (1), but in recent years many will acquire the label of chronic fatigue syndrome [CFS] or fibromyalgia.

The literature of CFS is expanding rapidly. Specialist reviews have appeared concerning virology, immunology, psychiatry, epidemiology and treatment. This paper will consider the wider social and cultural aspects of the condition. There has been a tendency to neglect these aspects of CFS in favor of biomedical explanations, in the hope that some new discovery arising out of immunology or virology will explain the enigma of CFS. I shall argue that an understanding of the cultural background to CFS is equally pertinent.

A word of caution is in order given the controversial subject of this paper. There are two aspects to CFS. The first is an operationally-defined condition, that can be measured and studied. We and other groups are making progress in determining the epidemiology of CFS in primary care using the conventional methods of epidemiological research. However, such research will not shed light on the second problem of CFS. This is the

Simon Wessely, MA, BM, BCh, MSc, MD, MRCP, MRCPsych, is Senior Lecturer in Psychological Medicine, King's College Hospital Medical School and Institute of Psychiatry and Consultant Psychiatrist, King's College and Maudsley Hospital, Denmark Hill, London, United Kingdom SE5 9RS.

[Haworth co-indexing entry note]: "Social and Cultural Aspects of Chronic Fatigue Syndrome." Wessely, Simon. Co-published simultaneously in the *Journal of Musculoskeletal Pain* (The Haworth Medical Press, an imprint of The Haworth Press, Inc.) Vol. 3, No. 2, 1995, pp. 111-122; and: *Fibromyalgia, Chronic Fatigue Syndrome, and Repetitive Strain Injury: Current Concepts in Diagnosis, Management, Disability, and Health Economics* (ed: Andrew Chalmers et al.) The Haworth Medical Press, an imprint of The Haworth Press, Inc., 1995, pp. 111-122. Multiple copies of this article/chapter may be purchased from The Haworth Document Delivery Center [1-800-3-HAWORTH; 9:00 a.m. - 5:00 p.m. (EST)].

© 1995 by The Haworth Press, Inc. All rights reserved.

111

belief, whether self- or doctor-generated, that one is suffering from an illness with that label. Thus, patients are appearing in increasing numbers who believe, often with passion and conviction, that they suffer from chronic fatigue and immune deficiency syndrome (CFIDS) in the USA, or myalgic encephalomyelitis (ME) in the United Kingdom. I have argued the importance of distinguishing these two distinct themes (2). Our group will present data showing that many of those who fulfil criteria for CFS in the community who are not seeking help attribute their illness to other causes. On the other hand, many of those who do believe that they have the condition do not fulfil the criteria.

As an epidemiologist, I know that a person has CFS only if they fulfil operational criteria. As an observer of the social scene, I also know that ME or CFIDS is defined by the sufferers themselves. Hence, for this paper, a person has ME or CFIDS simply if that is what they believe is wrong with them. Untold confusion has arisen from the failure to distinguish between an operationally-defined epidemiological construct and a social belief system. This essay concerns the latter and not the former.

PSYCHIATRIC DISORDER AND CFS

Wherever CFS patients are studied, and however they are studied, psychological morbidity is conspicuous by its presence. It is a matter of regret that each generation of physicians appears to need to discover this afresh, and that such observations continue to inspire the same futile "organic versus psychological" polemics (1). Once again, numerous studies confirm that the majority of those seen in specialist centers and primary care with a chief complaint of chronic fatigue fulfill operational criteria for a psychiatric disorder. The consequence of physical disease cannot alone account for the clinical features of CFS (3,4).

These findings do not mean that psychiatric disorder causes CFS, or that CFS and psychiatric disorder are one and the same. One must not forget that psychiatric disorder in general, and depression in particular, are heterogenous concepts. The possibility that both CFS and psychiatric disorder have a common origin in disturbances of cerebral function now attracts considerable attention (5), and some evidence is emerging of neurobiological differences between the subgroup of CFS patients without depression and both normal and depressed controls.

A more appropriate conclusion is that the current acrimonious debate over the relationship between CFS and psychiatric disorder based solely on comparisons of operational criteria is unhelpful. Chronic fatigue syndrome and psychiatric disorder go together. It is inevitable because of the way both concepts have been constructed, the similarities of the criteria and the measures used to define them. Operational criteria will be unable to make a complete distinction between CFS and psychiatric disorders. To understand these differences once must turn to the role of social and cultural factors.

A flavor of these differences comes from the popular literature on chronic fatigue syndrome. Take the issue of personality and vulnerability to CFS. Sufferers are often characterized as perfectionists and over-achievers. One sufferer told the journalist that "until my symptoms started I gave 120% to every aspect of my life." Hence when she picked up an infection, "instead of resting I just carried on" (6). Sufferers are particu-larly prone to be overactive, unlikely to take things easy, "the last people to take time off work for no good reason" (7). "It seemed like a bad bout of flu from which [as usual] I did not allow myself proper time to recover" (8). Sufferers "work until they drop, whilst everyone else creeps to bed with the slightest headache or sniffle . . . lazy people don't get ME" (9).

The cultural purpose of these stereotypes is to separate CFS from another stereotype–those patients who do none of these things–by implica-tion those who do take time off work for no good reason, who do creep to bed with the slightest sniffle–psychiatric patients. The current President of the ME Association stated that one of the distinctive differences between ME sufferers and depressives is that those with ME are highly-motivated achievers, "they almost have too much will power, whereas depressives have virtually none" (10). If psychiatric disorder is seen in these Victorian terms, it is not surprising that it is something to avoid. Hence the descrip-tions of overachieving, duty-driven victims of CFS is one strategy for countering any suggestion of a psychological origin to symptoms.

THE SEARCH FOR VALIDATION

At the heart of CFS is the rejection of any form of psychological causation or treatment. In the first newsletter of the ME Action Campaign, Claire Francis, the President of the Campaign and without doubt the most famous sufferer from CFS in Britain, wrote that "psychiatry is the dustbin of the medical profession" (11). Hence few sufferers come anywhere near a psychiatrist. Being referred to a psychiatrist is "being blackballed" (12), "being imprisoned for a crime I didn't do" (13), or being on trial (14). Courtroom analogies are apt, since the atmosphere surrounding CFS is now an adversarial one, accompanied by a rhetoric of struggle and injus-tice–a typical headline is, "Justice for the neglected and maligned suffer-ers of ME" (15). Others speak of bitterness, anger, and hate. The accusa-tion is not just that the sufferer is guilty of being depressed, or of having a psychiatric disorder, but of not being ill at all–of having an imaginary disease.

Here is another tragedy of CFS. Many doctors do indeed equate psychological disorder with unreal disorder. The reluctance to accept suffering perceived as of psychological origin as genuine, is shared, and often initiated, by the medical profession. A doctor agreed that it is important that psychiatric patients are separated from ME because "some neurotic patients devalue the tales of genuine sufferers" (16). Another is quoted as telling a medical conference that "ME is an imaginary disease . . . for which the best treatment is psychiatric" (17). A recent article on chronic Lyme disease talked about the difficulties faced by patients in their dealing with doctors–"some were even considered malingerers. Many were referred to psychiatrists when their medical physicians lost faith in the validity of their patients' complaints" (18). Doctors thus share many of the prejudices of the CFS sufferer–psychiatrists treat imaginary, malingered or non-existent diseases.

The consequences of this lack of validation are many and grievous. One sufferer was refused sickness insurance benefit because his policy excluded depression, of which he had a past history. His claim to be now suffering from ME was rejected, although he was informed that this decision would be changed if a test for ME were to be developed and he tested positive (19). Hence sufferers cannot literally afford to be depressed. It is the search for validation that underlies the drive to find a test for CFS, and the rejoicing that greets each such claim. As one sufferer wrote, "the difference between a crazed neurotic and a seriously ill person is simply a test" (20). These views are understandable, since in the absence of acceptable tests or physical signs, onlookers find it harder to accept the reality of distress. The patient rarely looks sick. Sufferer after sufferer note how outsiders make comments, such as "well, you don't look sick–you look great" (21). "My skin is clear and tanned. I don't have a plaster cast on a broken leg . . . people say 'you look so well' " (22).

Similar observations have been made concerning chronic pain. Both fatigue and pain are private experiences to which no one else has access. In an insightful paper, aptly called "The Pilgrimage of Pain," Reid and colleagues (23) noted the problems encountered by RSI sufferers in their search for validity–endlessly shuttling between the company doctor accusing them of malingering, and the trade union doctor with an equal and opposite aversion to recognizing any psychological distress at all. Without a test, not just the CFS patient, but also the fibromyalgia and RSI sufferer, exist on the margins of sickness and disability.

WHY A VIRUS
[OR IMMUNE DEFECT, OR ALLERGY . . .]?

Why have there been such efforts to find a microbiological cause of CFS, and so many mutually exclusive claims of success over the years? It is true that many patients give a history of an initial "viral" illness. Nevertheless, with the exception of recent work demonstrating beyond doubt that the Epstein-Barr virus is indeed associated with a true post-infectious fatigue syndrome (24), proof that CFS is associated with either a post or persistent viral state is far from compelling.

One reason, beyond the scope of this paper, is methodological. Of more relevance are the social and cultural factors. The concept of an external agent is a familiar one for both doctor and patient. The external nature of the attribution made by the chronically fatigued patient seen in hospital practice has certain consequences, irrespective of its accuracy. External attribution may protect the patient from the stigma of being labelled psychiatrically disordered–"the victim of a germ infection is therefore blameless" (25). In the context of CFS "to attribute the continuing symptoms to persistence of a "physical" disease is a mechanism that carries the least threat to a person's self-esteem" (26). The absence of guilt and the preservation of self-esteem, even in the presence of mood disorder, has been noted in post-infectious fatigue syndromes (27).

What the many popular explanations have in common is that they are external to the patient, and are not accompanied by accusations of moral weakness or blame (28). CFS has been claimed to be due to viruses, electromagnetic radiation, geopathic stress, dental amalgam, candida, food allergy, pesticides, antibiotics, immunization and so on. This is well caught in the media writing on CFS. A newspaper headline expressed this view in its clearest form : "Virus research doctors finally prove shirkers really are sick" (29), while a Times piece was titled, "Fatigue blamed on virus: Malingering disease proved genuine" (30). A recent review of a self-help book noted "an infection is respectable. It has none of the stigma of a psychologically induced illness, which implies weakness or lack of moral fibre" (31). It is also a popular explanation for disease in the English-speaking world. Finally, the rise of HIV has meant that the concept of a deadly virus that affects the immune system is now one deeply embedded in popular consciousness. Direct analogies between AIDS and CFS are common–the name adopted by the most vigorous of the campaigning organizations in the USA–the Chronic Fatigue and Immune Deficiency Syndrome–is a conscious attempt to draw upon the experience of AIDS.

DOES IT MATTER?

At present the prognosis for those who have acquired, by whatever means, the label of CFS or its local equivalents, is poor. Behan and Behan (32), who have perhaps the most extensive experience of CFS in this country, wrote that "most cases do not improve, give up their work and become permanent invalids, incapacitated by excessive fatigue and myalgia," confirmed by systematic follow-ups of those referred to an immunology or an infectious disease clinic (33,34). The main association of poor prognosis was the strength of belief in an exclusively physical cause for symptoms (34,35).

Much of the current information on CFS may also adversely influence prognosis. Current literature on CFS is frequently gloomy in tone, with a tendency to use "worst case" examples for publicity purposes. The first President of the ME Association and its first medical advisor used the same words–the disease has "an alarming tendency to chronicity" (36,37). Those who champion the disease often insist that an essential clinical feature of the disease is "a prolonged relapsing course lasting years or decades" (38). Newspapers and magazines frequently call the disease incurable. How much is this perception based on clinical reality, and how much does it influence that reality?

The climate of opinion and controversy surrounding CFS means that the sufferer is frequently caught in a trap. The treatments suggested by a model of CFS as a unitary condition, the sole consequence of a single physical agent, are straightforward, simple to explain, free of stigma and moral implications. As yet, few appear to work. On the other hand, other strategies, based on a more complex model, involving either psychological or behavioral interventions, are far from value-free. All of this is magnified in the light of the controversy surrounding CFS. In this climate accepting any treatment other than those based on the single disease/external agent model is fraught with difficulty. The hostility towards psychological distress, perceived as it is as synonymous with low moral fiber and blame, permeates treatment and outcome. Psychiatrists are seen as having little or no role in the management of CFS. In the CFS literature, often the good psychiatrist is the one who finds nothing wrong and declares the sufferer psychologically normal.

REST AND THE TREATMENT OF CFS

At present, the mainstay of management in CFS is rest. A nurse with CFS advises others, "Always remember, until an exciting medical announcement is made, that there is no one drug to cure ME. The only cure is rest and keeping the affected parts of the body rigid so as to improve the body's defenses" (39). Similar sentiments were expressed in a magazine–"the only hope is that one day some substance will be isolated that has the power to zap the ME virus," and until then "the most doctors can do is to advise patients to rest, and wait for the ME to go away" (40). The familiar Victorian metaphor of the supply and demand of energy reappears frequently–"use energy at a slower rate than you make it" (41). The treatment frequently comes back to that mainstay of the Victorian approach to neurasthenia, the rest cure. An American self-help book heads a section with the title "Rest, Rest and More Rest" (42), and discusses "Aggressive rest therapy," as does an English self-help title (43).

Although there is no doubting the good faith behind such advice, its long-term wisdom is open to question, and is at odds with most medical teaching. Despite this, rest is one part of the spectrum of avoidance behaviors that characterize much of the popular management of chronic fatigue syndrome. A frequent theme is the need to avoid various agents, ranging from immunizations and pollution to a variety of foods and even sunlight that may affect the illness. In its most extreme form CFS overlaps with such Western cultural syndromes as multiple chemical sensitivity or total allergy syndrome, where lives are ruined by fearful anticipation and avoidance of most forms of environmental stimulation.

Why is rest so popular? One reason is that it appears to work. Rest is an effective short-term strategy for dealing with acute fatigue, particularly after acute infection, which is so often the trigger for chronic fatigue syndrome. For most subjects, such rest is only used as a short-term coping strategy, and the vast majority are able to resume normal activity. However, recovery from viral infection is almost certainly normally distributed, and some may experience a prolonged, and inexplicable, period of ill health. Attempts to resume previous levels of activity may continue to be difficult during this period, and result in a resurgence of symptoms.

Many have noted that many chronic sufferers initially adopted a vigorous program of exercise–there are numerous anecdotal reports of chronic sufferers with a previous history of an abrupt return to dramatic physical activity. There are several reasons for this. First, this author's experience is that CFS patients seen in the clinic are frequently particularly fit and athletic. Such patients would be at risk of rapid physical deconditioning after a period of enforced rest. Furthermore, personality and lifestyle factors may also suggest that the same people are also likely to adopt overly aggressive early attempts at exercise. I have already discussed the popular stereotype reinforced by the CFS organizations that sufferers are particularly prone to be overactive, unlikely to take things easy and so on [vide supra]. Many have tried to "exercise away" their fatigue, and hence carried out activity that might be excessive in the light of their current, but not previous, fitness.

What are the consequences? They need little elaboration to the audience of this paper. One general practitioner who is a sufferer and author of a popular self-help guide has written "prolonged bed rest . . . should be advised with great care in the long-term cases, who may then become trapped in a vicious circle of immobility and weakness, and become almost bedridden" (7). The consequences of lack of physical activity, and the changes in the neuromuscular system that result, have been known to clinicians for many years and will not be elaborated in detail. Rest as a coping strategy is thus of short-term benefit to those with acute fatigue syndromes, but in the long-term is harmful.

THE SOCIAL PURPOSE OF CFS

One purpose of CFS is to give legitimacy to distress that would otherwise be unacceptable to the patient, relative, employer, doctor and insurer. This has many benefits. I have pointed out how badly doctors can treat the patient perceived to have a psychological origin to their distress. This can be avoided when the label of CFS is seen to indicate a physical, and hence, blameless, etiology.

The second purpose may be to allow the sufferer to make necessary changes in their life without stigma. The self-help literature on CFS is equally full of wide-ranging suggestions for changes in lifestyle. A typical book (44) includes not only the usual advice on diet, rest, exercise, candida, stress and work, but also sections on the power of prayer, attitudes, the need to love oneself, and a section discussing the relative merits of holidays in the mountains or the Mediterranean, just as the neurasthenia texts discussed the merits of the different European spas.

Sufferers are urged to alter their lifestyle by placing their own personal well-being, comfort and happiness at the center of their concern. A sufferer must accept an inability to live at the same pace as previously, but this can lead to moral and spiritual benefits. Self-worth is "not measured by being busy, earning money or even being good at anything" (45). Of the patients studied by Norma Ware in Boston, nearly half had undergone a transformation of lifestyles as a result of CFS, which they declared to be painful, but ultimately positive (21). In this country, an actor told a newspaper that ME had "been like a gift, as though it was sent to sort my life out . . . My life has taken a completely different direction" (46). One

American sufferer found that CFS led her to consider "better ways to feel, think and relate" and to address the chronic stresses of her life, which were responsible for the depletion of her immune system (47). Another sufferer wrote that as a result of ME, "I have tried to use the time positively to make changes I accept were overdue," going on to describe reassessment of work, relationships and so on (48). A doctor with ME became a changed woman, seeing "a value in going for a walk on her own. She feels no guilt about enjoying herself or taking time off to relax" (49).

As well as permitting changes to lifestyle, CFS serves as a conduit for social concerns, expressed via the metaphor of illness (2). Neurasthenia was frequently blamed on the unwelcome features of contemporary life (1). Contemporaries such as George Beard blamed the unwelcome intrusion of modern technology and business practice for the rise of the new disease of nervous exhaustion. Others blamed neurasthenia on the "dust, and whistling, noisy pandemonium, smoke and bad air of the city" (50). Neurasthenia texts struck a balance between the language of the current scientific discourse, and concerns and language that were meaningful to the lay reader. Much of this was conveyed by metaphors. These could be drawn from business life and commerce–"The strenuous man of business knows well the significance of an overdraft in his bank account, and does not treat it so lightly as an overdraft on his nerve center balance" (51) or alternatively, from popular science–"the storage battery has been discharged rapidly or for too long a time" (52). Similarly, the modern CFS "sufferer should treat her energy resources as if they were money in the bank, and be careful not to overdraw" (53). Alternatively, they must have batteries that are either flat (54), unable to hold their charge (45), or in need of recharging (55).

An individual's responsibility for neurasthenia then and CFS now is thus restricted to the relatively blameless [and indeed praiseworthy] habit of overwork, of struggling on beyond the limits of what is physiologically tolerable. If overwork summarizes the individual's role in acquiring CFS, that of society is summarized by "overload." According to Beard (56), the unwelcome features of contemporary life which caused neurasthenia did so by creating an "overload," or "overloaded system." The same concepts have surfaced in the context of CFS/ME. Articles are frequently entitled "the ME Generation"–one began with the question "What is modern life doing to us?" (57). Another popular magazine suggests that "ME is very much a disease of our time–an attack on the immune system exacerbated by stress, pressure and the demands of twentieth century life" (58). ME is "an overload disease unique to this century" (59). Nowadays, the overload is due to pesticides, allergies, chemicals, neurotoxins, antibiotics, over-refined diet, pollution, electromagnetic radiation, candida and so on. CFS is due to the "sickness of the planet" (59).

Will CFS go the same way as neurasthenia? I suspect not, for three reasons. First, the rise of modern neurobiological research has meant that previous boundaries between psychiatric and physical disease are dissolving, although not as rapidly as one would like. There is every prospect of new insights being gained into fundamental central mechanisms underlying CFS. Second, once an agnostic, I am inclined to believe that an entity called CFS can be located in the community, although I suspect that, like fibromyalgia, it will be the arbitrary end of a spectrum of fatigue and exhaustion. Finally, the changes in the relationship between the modern patient and doctor have been so profound, with the balance shifting from the former to the latter, that academic arguments about the status of CFS are becoming overtaken by events. Whether it exists or not, it is here to stay.

REFERENCES

1. Wessely S: The history of chronic fatigue syndrome. Chronic Fatigue Syndrome. Edited by S Straus. New York; Mark Dekker, 1994, pp. 41-82.

2. Wessely S: Neurasthenia and chronic fatigue syndrome: theory and practice. Transcultural Psychiatric Review 31: 173-209, 1994.

3. Wood G, Bentall R, Gopfert M, Edwards R: A comparative psychiatric assessment of patients with chronic fatigue syndrome and muscle disease. Psychological Medicine 21: 619-628, 1991.

4. Katon W, Buchwald D, Simon G, Russo J, Mease P: Psychiatric illness in chronic fatigue syndrome. J General Internal Medicine 6: 277-285, 1991.

5. Bearn J, Wessely S: The neurobiology of chronic fatigue syndrome. Eur J Clinical Investigation 24: 79-90, 1994.

6. Macdonald K: Why perfectionists are most at risk from ME. Daily Mail Sept 28th 1993.

7. Shepherd C: Living with ME: a Self-Help Guide. London, Heinemann, 1989.

8. Roeber J: Industry of Anxiety. Vogue, August 1989, 178-179.

9. Bragg P: Kilroy was here. Interaction 3, Autumn 1989, 503.

10. Dowsett E: quoted in Stacey S. "Tired and Tested." Harpers & Queen, Oct 1990.

11. Francis C: A Beginning. Interaction 1, 1988.

12. Conant S: Living With Chronic Fatigue. Taylor; Dallas; 1990.

13. Gardner K: Interaction 1; Winter 1988.

14. Hartnell L: British Medical Journal 10th June 1989; 1577-1578.

15. Field E: Justice for the neglected and maligned sufferers of ME. Guardian, 7th August 1990.

16. Timbs O: Postviral puzzle. Observer, 2nd August 1987.

17. Herbert V: cited in Steincamp J. Overload: Beating M.E. Fontana, London, 1989, p. 5.

18. Burrascano J: The overdiagnosis of Lyme Disease. J Am Med Assoc 270:2682, 1993.

19. Stopp C: ME sufferers forced to battle with insurers. Independent on Sunday 27th June 1993.

20. Jeffries T: The Mile High Staircase. Auckland, Hodder & Stoughton, 1982.

21. Ware N: Society, mind and body in chronic fatigue syndrome: an anthropological view. Chronic fatigue syndrome. Edited by A Kleinman, S Straus. Wiley, Chichester (CIBA Foundation Symposium 173); 1993, pp. 62-82.

22. Berrett J: Condemned to live a lonely life. Guardian July 6th 1991.

23. Reid J, Ewan C, Lowy E: Pilgrimage of pain: the illness experiences of women with repetition strain injury and the search for credibility. Social Science Med 32:601-612, 1991.

24. White P, Thomas J, Amess J, Grover S, Kangro H, Clare A: A fatigue syndrome following infectious mononucleosis: 1: the existence of the syndrome. Submitted.

25. Helman C: Feed a cold and starve a fever. Culture, Medicine & Psychiatry 7; 107-137, 1978.

26. Katz B, Andiman W: Chronic Fatigue Syndrome. J Pediatrics 113; 944-947, 1978.

27. Imboden J, Canter A, Cluff L: Brucellosis.III. Psychologic aspects of delayed convalescence. Arch Intern Med 103: 406-414, 1959.

28. Abbey S: Somatization, illness attribution and the sociocultural psychiatry of chronic fatigue syndrome. Chronic fatigue syndrome. Edited by A Kleinman, S Straus. Wiley, Chichester (CIBA Foundation Symposium 173); pp. 238-261.

29. Hodgkinson N: Virus research doctors finally prove shirkers really are sick. Sunday Times, 25th January 1987.

30. Anon. The Times, Jan 2 1988.

31. Seagrove J: The ME Generation. Guardian May 19 1989.

32. Behan P, Behan W: The Postviral Fatigue Syndrome. CRC Critical Reviews in Neurobiology 42: 157-178, 1988.

33. Hinds G, McCluskey D: A retrospective study of the chronic fatigue syndrome. Proc R Coll Physicians Edin 23:10-14, 1993.

34. Sharpe M, Hawton K, Seagroatt V, Pasvol G: Follow up of patients with fatigue presenting to an infectious diseases clinic. Br Med J 305:347-352, 1992.

35. Wilson A, Hickie I, Lloyd A, Hadzi-Pavlovic D, Boughton C, Dwyer J, Wakefield D: Longitudinal study of the outcome of chronic fatigue syndrome. Br Med J 308: 756-760, 1994.

36. Ramsay M: Introduction to Shepherd, C. Living with ME; A Self Help Guide. Heinemann, London, 1989.

37. Smith D: Myalgic encephalomyelitis. 1989 Members Reference Book. Royal College of General Practitioners: Sabre Crown Publishing, London, 1989, pp. 247-250.

38. Dowsett E, Welsby P: Conversation piece. Postgrad Med J 68:63-65, 1992.

39. Dainty E. M.E. and I: Nursing Standard 84: 49-50, 1988.

40. Hodgkinson L: M.E.–the mystery disease. Women's Journal, November 1988.

41. Holford N: ME. Report of the Assistant Masters and Mistresses Association, Sept 1989, 12-13.

42. Feiden K: Hope and Help for Chronic Fatigue Syndrome. Prentice Hall, New York, 1990.

43. Franklin M, Sullivan J: The New Mystery Fatigue Epidemic. M.E. What is it? Have you got it? How to get better. Century, London, 1989.

44. Dawes B, Downing D: Why M.E.? A Guide to Combatting Post-Viral Illness. Grafton, London, 1989.

45. MacIntyre A: ME: Post-Viral Fatigue Syndrome: How to Live with It. London, Unwin; 1989.

46. My battle with "devil" illness, by Bergerac star Sean; Daily Mail, 8 Sept 1990.

47. D Patrick Miller. My healing journey through chronic fatigue. Yoga Journal Nov/Dec 1992.

48. Berrett J: Condemned to live a lonely life. Guardian July 6th 1991.

49. When the drive band snaps. Hampstead and Highgate Gazette, August 5th, 1988.

50. Ely T: Neurasthenia as modified by modern conditions, and their prevention. Journal American Medical Association 47; 1816-1819, 1906.

51. Hughes C: Psychiatry and Neuriatry in the Medical Press. Alienist and Neurologist 27: 452-460, 1906.

52. Pershing H: The treatment of neurasthenia. Medical News 84;637-640, 1904.

53. "Postviral Fatigue Syndrome." In: The Manual of Family Health. Royal College of Nursing. Little, Brown: London, 1992; pp. 489-490.

54. Stacey S: Tired and Tested. Harpers & Queen, Oct 1990.

55. Millenson J: ME: An Alternative View. Interaction 9, Spring 1992.

56. Beard G: American Nervousness. New York: G.P. Putnam's, 1881.

57. The ME Generation. Sunday Telegraph Weekend Magazine, Jan 22nd 1989.

58. Flett K: Why M.E.? Arena, March 1990.

59. Steincamp J: Overload: Beating M.E. Fontana, London, 1989.

60. The Internal Athlete. MS. Volume II, No 6. May/June 1992.

Approaches to RSI in the United Kingdom

Paul A. Reilly

SUMMARY. Objectives: To review the factors influencing the current epidemic of work-related upper limb pain in the United Kingdom, and to discuss the role of Medicine and Law in its genesis and perpetuation.

Methods: Informed observation.

Findings: The epidemic has a multifactorial etiology. It is best viewed as a complex psychosocial phenomenon, with historical precedents in writers' and telegraphists' cramps of the last century. The unhelpful interaction of doctors, lawyers, the media, trade unions and society as a whole has been to the detriment of sufferers.

Conclusions: Greater understanding of the complex nature of chronic pain and the avoidance of confrontation and litigation are to be encouraged if the United Kingdom [UK] is not to follow the same ruinous path as Australia a decade ago.

KEYWORDS. Overuse syndrome, cumulative trauma disorder, occupational neurosis, upper limb pain, repetitive strain injury

INTRODUCTION

The United Kingdom [UK] is currently experiencing a dramatic rise in the incidence of work-related upper limb disorder [also called repetitive

Paul A. Reilly, MB ChB, MRCP[UK], is Consultant in Rheumatology and Pain Management, Frimley Park NHS Trust Hospital, Portsmouth Road, Camberley, Surrey, England GU16 5UJ.

[Haworth co-indexing entry note]: "Approaches to RSI in the United Kingdom." Reilly, Paul A. Co-published simultaneously in the *Journal of Musculoskeletal Pain* (The Haworth Medical Press, an imprint of The Haworth Press, Inc.) Vol. 3, No. 2, 1995, pp. 123-125; and: *Fibromyalgia, Chronic Fatigue Syndrome, and Repetitive Strain Injury: Current Concepts in Diagnosis, Management, Disability, and Health Economics* (ed: Andrew Chalmers et al.) The Haworth Medical Press, an imprint of The Haworth Press, Inc., 1995, pp. 123-125. Multiple copies of this article/chapter may be purchased from The Haworth Document Delivery Center [1-800-3-HAWORTH; 9:00 a.m. - 5:00 p.m. (EST)].

© 1995 by The Haworth Press, Inc. All rights reserved.

123

strain injury, RSI]. The overall pattern is proving very similar to that of Australia in the 1970s and 1980s. A failure to understand the complex and multifactorial basis of chronic pain syndromes on the part of medical and paramedical practitioners is helping to promote and perpetuate the epidemic. So are the adversarial legal system, sensationalism in the media, and faulty beliefs in those experiencing upper limb discomfort. We have not learned [yet] from the Australian experience, and the epidemic is still on the increase.

Britain has an unenviable record of upper limb pain in workers. In the late 18th and early 19th centuries, there were epidemics of writers' cramp in clerks, and telegraphists' cramp in telegraph operators. Both were attributed to new technology, the steel-nibbed pen and the telegraph pad, respectively. Both epidemics were closely scrutinized for the effect of physical factors: hours worked, length of service, workplace design, type of equipment used, age, body build, etc. In the end, it was concluded that temperament and personality were the main determinants of susceptibility to the problem, and that the illnesses were largely psychosomatic.

FROM EMPLOYEE TO INVALID

In the UK, RSI mainly affects younger females, working either in a secretarial capacity or in processing and manufacturing. The use, or rather overuse, of a keyboard is often blamed in white-collar industries. These are often large, public-sector organizations, such as the Inland Revenue service, the British Broadcasting Corporation [BBC], and the Post Office. Also affected are national clearing banks [especially among check encoders], newspaper and other media offices [one of the few areas where males have featured in the problem], and companies with large numbers of secretaries, such as in the bigger legal and accountancy firms. A major poultry processing company has recently lost a significant legal case, and expects more than a hundred other claims to follow. As in Australia, the self-employed rarely present with repetitive strain injury.

The progression from transient ache in the hand, wrist or forearm to a chronic, disabling pain syndrome often begins with the primary care physician, who, by extrapolating from previous patients with typical de Quervains disease or lateral epicondylitis, will diagnose tenosynovitis, tennis elbow, carpal tunnel syndrome, or increasingly repetitve strain injury. This first diagnostic term is often very difficult to overcome subsequently. The employee is signed off work and advised to rest the limb completely for 2-4 weeks. Analgesics, splints or physiotherapy may be prescribed, but the problem persists or worsens. The company Occupational Health Physician, perhaps on the instructions of the personnel department, may not allow the employee to return to work until fully fit, there being few opportunities for light duties during a period of national economic recession. Symptoms may be reinforced by reading leaflets from the government-run Health and Safety Executive and from self-help groups, such as the RSI Association. The employee's trade union may now become involved, advising litigation on the grounds of negligence by management. There follows visits to lawyers, then "expert" medical opinions from doctors retained by both sides, and eventually a stressful legal case in the High Court. This whole process may take years, and there is little chance of successful rehabilitation in the meantime.

The considerable hassle, strain and time required for contentious medico-legal work in such an imprecise area of medicine is persuading many erudite clinicians to avoid getting involved. Therefore, the number of expert witnesses willing to see claimants and attend Court is falling. Yet, every successful claim publicized in the popular press and trade journals acts as a spur to other workers with upper limb pain to proceed to litigation.

FUTURE TRENDS

Gradually, a better awareness of the nature of the problem is developing in industry. Early sympathetic management, on-the-job rehabilitation programs, and a graduated re-entry to normal working practice can be offered. Initial results are encouraging. Avoiding confrontation and the adversarial British legal system are certainly important, as is better education of doctors, physiotherapists, and employees on the nature of pain and its variable relationship to work, injury and disease.

CONCLUSION

The novel technologies of today become standard tools of tomorrow. The temptation to blame the steel-nibbed pen, telegraph or word processor for upper limb discomfort may well be strong when the user is uncertain of the effect the new tool will have on such intangibles as job security and satisfaction. While some workers will always seek the path of least resistance away from a situation of pressure and stress, we should recall that previous epidemics of work-related arm pain subsided in due course. Either RSI will follow that pattern, or it will reappear in the future with yet another new name. Our job as doctors is to ensure that workers are protected as much from ignorance as from negligence.

The Direct Costs
of Fibromyalgia Treatment:
Comparison with Rheumatoid Arthritis
and Osteoarthritis

Robert W. Simms
Leslie Cahill
Mark Prashker
Robert F. Meenan

KEYWORDS. Direct costs, treatment, fibromyalgia syndrome

Rising health care costs are one of the cornerstones of the national debate on health care reform since medical care costs have been rising at over twice the rate of inflation yearly for the past decade. Despite the fact that fibromyalgia is a common chronic condition (1), little is known of the direct or indirect costs associated with the care of patients with fibromyal-

---

Robert W. Simms, MD, is affiliated with Boston University School of Medicine, Boston, MA.

Leslie Cahill, MPH, and Mark Prashker, MD, MPH, are affiliated with Boston University School of Medicine and Boston Veteran's Administration Medical Center, Boston, MA.

Robert F. Meenan, MD, MPH, MBA, is affiliated with Boston University School of Public Health, Boston, MA.

Address correspondence to: Robert W. Simms, MD, Arthritis Center, Boston University School of Medicine, 71 East Concord Street, Boston, MA 02118.

[Haworth co-indexing entry note]: "The Direct Costs of Fibromyalgia Treatment: Comparison with Rheumatoid Arthritis and Osteoarthritis." Simms, Robert W. et al. Co-published simultaneously in the *Journal of Musculoskeletal Pain* (The Haworth Medical Press, an imprint of The Haworth Press, Inc.) Vol. 3, No. 2, 1995, pp. 127-132; and: *Fibromyalgia, Chronic Fatigue Syndrome, and Repetitive Strain Injury: Current Concepts in Diagnosis, Management, Disability, and Health Economics* (ed: Andrew Chalmers et al.) The Haworth Medical Press, an imprint of The Haworth Press, Inc., 1995, pp. 127-132. Multiple copies of this article/chapter may be purchased from The Haworth Document Delivery Center [1-800-3-HAWORTH; 9:00 a.m. - 5:00 p.m. (EST)].

© 1995 by The Haworth Press, Inc. All rights reserved.   *127*

gia syndrome. Also, it remains unknown how fibromyalgia syndrome treatment costs compare to the costs of treating the two other most common rheumatic conditions seen in rheumatology practices, namely osteoarthritis and rheumatoid arthritis.

To compare the direct costs of treating the three most common rheumatic conditions [fibromyalgia syndrome, osteoarthritis, and rheumatoid arthritis], we utilized a cost of treatment index [CTI] (2). The CTI focuses on a given disease and examines the number of inputs utilized to treat the disease for a fixed time period and compares the cost of treating that disease over time. The CTI has two principle advantages over the medical care price index [MCPI], the traditional method of measuring changes in health care costs: 1. the CTI eliminates sampling bias inherent in the MCPI, and 2. it reflects quality changes and the introduction of new products and techniques which are not captured well in the MCPI.

METHODS

We obtained one year of utilization and charge information for all patients seen in 1986 and in 1991 with fibromyalgia syndrome, osteoarthritis and rheumatoid arthritis at the Boston University Arthritis Center, a large, academic group practice with a special interest in fibromyalgia syndrome. Demographic, disease duration and medication information was obtained from the medical record of each patient. Charge data were converted to cost data using institutional cost/charge ratios and were multiplied by utilization data to obtain cost data for each patient. The cost data were then aggregated by patient diagnosis. The four principle components of cost included: 1. office visits, 2. medications, 3. laboratory tests, and 4. imaging studies. Office visit costs reflected the mean cost for physician office visits for all patients within a given disease category. Medication cost data was obtained from the medical record and from Redbook wholesale charge information and included both prescription and non-prescription medications. Where appropriate, we assumed that medications listed in the medical record were continued for the calendar year studied. Laboratory costs include the cost of all non-imaging laboratory tests. Imaging costs included those for plain x-ray films, computerized tomography [CT] scans, and magnetic resonance imaging [MRI] studies. Not assessed were non-prescribed treatments or non-medication therapies such as physical therapy, chiropractic manipulation, psychotherapy or acupuncture. To ensure that changes in cost over time were not due to case mix changes, we adjusted the data for age and disease duration.

RESULTS

A total of 210 patients with fibromyalgia, 220 with osteoarthritis and 136 with rheumatoid arthritis were studied. Table 1 shows the population characteristics. The mean age, % female and disease durations for each of the disorders, indicate that the population studied was similar to that of previous descriptions for these conditions (3-5).

Figure 1 indicates how the costs for each of the four cost categories compares for fibromyalgia, osteoarthritis, and rheumatoid arthritis for both 1986 and 1991. It is evident medication costs account for the majority of treatment costs for each of the three diseases. Office visits, laboratory tests and imaging procedures contribute a much smaller proportion of the

TABLE 1. Population Characteristics

	Fibromyalgia	Osteoarthritis	Rheumatoid Arthritis
Disease Duration [yrs]	4.4 ± 3.3	5.8 ± 4.3	6.2 ± 3.9
% Female	92	65	69
Mean Age [yrs]	44 ± 11	62 ± 13	56 ± 16

FIGURE 1. Comparative direct costs for OA, RA and FMS in 1986 and 1991.

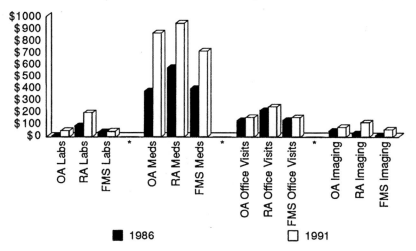

total treatment costs. Rheumatoid arthritis treatment costs are somewhat greater in all categories than either fibromyalgia or osteoarthritis. As one might expect, the laboratory costs for rheumatoid arthritis are greater than for osteoarthritis or fibromyalgia.

Figure 2 demonstrates the breakdown in medication costs for fibromyalgia from 1986 and 1991. Most of the cost of medication was attributable to three categories of medication: cyclobenzaprine, amitriptyline and nonsteroidal anti-inflammatory agents [NSAIDs]. Although the cost of medication increased within each medication category, the greatest increase in cost of medication in this five-year time period occurred in the NSAID category.

To assess how much control physicians can exert on medical care cost increases, we determined if increased costs represented increases in the numbers or types of tests and medications ordered by physicians or in the amount charged for these expenses. For fibromyalgia, increased costs were primarily due to price increases out of the control of physicians, particularly for medication, but also to a lesser extent laboratory and office visits. An exception was imaging in which there was a large increase in inputs due to the introduction of MRI between 1986 and 1991. As indicated in Figure 1, however, the proportion of total cost attributable to imaging for each of the disease categories was small.

FIGURE 2. Breakdown of medication costs for FMS in 1986 and 1991.

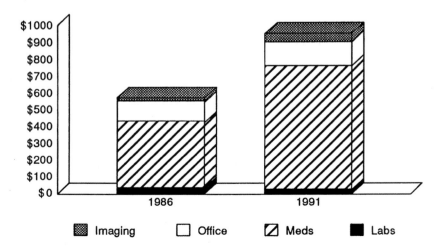

DISCUSSION

In this study, medications account for the principle direct cost of treating fibromyalgia, osteoarthritis and rheumatoid arthritis. Furthermore, increases in the cost of treatment from 1986 to 1991 were chiefly the result of increases in the cost of medications for each of the disorders under study. For fibromyalgia, with the exception of imaging, little change in inputs occurred from 1986 to 1991, indicating that increases in cost occurred chiefly as the result of increases in the price of inputs to care and not in the numbers or types of laboratory tests, medications, office visits, or imaging studies. Thus, a substantial proportion of the increase in the direct cost of treatment of fibromyalgia under the conditions studied was due to price increases in medications used to treat this syndrome.

The overall magnitude of the direct cost of treating fibromyalgia in this study was similar to osteoarthritis and rheumatoid arthritis. Since patients with fibromyalgia syndrome are likely to utilize treatments other than those included in this study [such as physical therapy and acupuncture] at rates which exceed those of patients with osteoarthritis and rheumatoid arthritis, our data likely underestimates the direct costs of treating fibromyalgia. The true cost of a disorder represents both direct and indirect costs [such as lost wages due to disability], and fibromyalgia syndrome, by some estimates, may produce rates of disability which approach that of rheumatoid arthritis (6). It is likely then that the overall cost of fibromyalgia, given its prevalence of approximately 2% of the adult United States population, is quite high.

The current debate on health care reform, has cost reduction as a cornerstone of virtually all proposed plans currently before Congress, since it is widely recognized that health care costs require some form of containment. We have shown in this study, that medication costs account for the largest proportion of total costs in treating these three common rheumatic conditions. Of interest is that over the time period under study, from 1986 to 1991, medication costs remained not only the largest single contributor to the cost of treatment but increased disproportionally when compared with cost components such as office visits, laboratory tests, and imaging procedures. Also of interest is the observation that the increase in cost attributable to medications was primarily the result of price increases, and not increases in the number of medications ordered by physicians. These data suggest that physicians are not ordering more medications to treat patients with fibromyalgia syndrome, rather the medications which they now utilize to treat patients cost more. It is also notable that NSAIDs, as a class of agents, account for the largest single increase in cost of treating fibromyalgia syndrome. The use of NSAIDs is particularly striking in view of their lack of efficacy in controlled trials of therapy in fibromyalgia syndrome (7,8). Reducing the use of NSAIDs in the treatment of fibromyalgia may be one way to reduce the direct costs of treating this condition.

In summary, medications constitute the principle direct cost of treating the most common rheumatic conditions: fibromyalgia syndrome, osteoarthritis and rheumatoid arthritis. For fibromyalgia, with the exception of imaging, little change in inputs occurred from 1986 to 1991, indicating that the substantial cost increases occurred chiefly as the result of increases in the prices of the medications. The overall magnitude of the cost of treatment of fibromyalgia appears to be similar to rheumatoid arthritis and osteoarthritis. Determining the full economic impact of fibromyalgia will require assessment of both indirect and direct economic costs.

REFERENCES

1. Wolfe F, Ross K, Anderson J, Russell IJ: The prevalence and characteristics of fibromyalgia in the general population. Arthritis Rheum 38: 19-28, 1995.

2. Prashker M, Cahill LA, Meenan RF: Rheumatology costs are increasing faster than inflation: results of a rheumatology cost of treatment index (RCTI). Arthritis Rheum 36: S65, 1993 (supplement).

3. Mankin HJ: Clinical features of osteoarthritis. Edited by WN Kelly, ED Harris, S Ruddy, CB Sledge. Textbook of Rheumatology. Fourth Ed. WB Saunders, Philadelphia, 1993, pp. 1374-1377.

4. Bennett RM (1993) The fibromyalgia syndrome: myofascial pain and chronic fatigue syndrome. Edited by WN Kelly, ED Harris, S Ruddy, CB Sledge. Textbook of Rheumatology. Fourth Ed. WB Saunders, Philadelphia, 1993, pp. 471-476.

5. Harris ED (1993) Clinical features of rheumatoid arthritis. Edited by WN Kelly, ED Harris, S Ruddy, CB Sledge. Textbook of Rheumatology. Fourth Ed. WB Saunders, Philadelphia, 1993, pp. 874-901.

6. Mason JH, Silverman SL, Weaver AL, Simms RW: The impact of fibromyalgia on multiple aspects of health status. Scand J Rheumatol 94: 33, 1992 (supplement).

7. Yunus MB, Masi AT, Aldag JC: Short-term effects of ibuprofen in primary fibromyalgia syndrome: a double blind, placebo controlled trial. J Rheumatol 16: 527-532, 1989.

8. Goldenberg DL, Felson DT, Dinerman H: A randomized controlled trial of amitriptyline and naproxen in the treatment of fibromyalgia syndrome. Arthritis Rheum 29: 1371-1377, 1986.

What Have Clinical Trials Taught Us About the Treatment of Fibromyalgia?

Simon Carette

SUMMARY. The treatment of fibromyalgia is generally unsatisfactory. Tricyclic agents and aerobic exercises have been the most extensively studied. In short-term clinical trials, they show favorable results in small proportions of patients. Their long-term efficacy, however, still remains to be demonstrated. Other treatment modalities, including cognitive-behavioral approaches, have been less extensively studied and therefore specific recommendations cannot be made. So far, no treatment has been shown to have any significant impact on the natural history of this condition.

The treatment of fibromyalgia is difficult and at times frustrating to both patient and physician. Complete remission is rare as reflected by long-term follow-up studies which indicate that 60 to 75 percent of patients remain symptomatic over the years, independent of the treatment received [Table 1] (1-6).

Various pharmacologic and non-pharmacologic treatment modalities for fibromyalgia have been proposed over the past 10 years. Those that have been studied in randomized controlled trials are included in Table 2.

The majority of these 32 trials can be criticized on various methodolog-

Simon Carette, MD, FRCPC, is Professor of Medicine and Head of the Department of Medicine, Centre Hospitalier de l'Université Laval.

Address correspondence to: Dr. Simon Carette, Centre Hospitalier de l'Université Laval, 2705 Boulevard Laurier, Ste-Foy P.Q., Canada G1V 4G2.

[Haworth co-indexing entry note]: "What Have Clinical Trials Taught Us About the Treatment of Fibromyalgia?" Carette, Simon. Co-published simultaneously in the *Journal of Musculoskeletal Pain* (The Haworth Medical Press, an imprint of The Haworth Press, Inc.) Vol. 3, No. 2, 1995, pp. 133-140; and: *Fibromyalgia, Chronic Fatigue Syndrome, and Repetitive Strain Injury: Current Concepts in Diagnosis, Management, Disability, and Health Economics* (ed: Andrew Chalmers et al.) The Haworth Medical Press, an imprint of The Haworth Press, Inc., 1995, pp. 133-140. Multiple copies of this article/chapter may be purchased from The Haworth Document Delivery Center [1-800-3-HAWORTH; 9:00 a.m. - 5:00 p.m. (EST)].

© 1995 by The Haworth Press, Inc. All rights reserved.

TABLE 1. Long-term follow-up studies of patients with fibromyalgia.

			n	Follow-up	% improved	% unchanged or worse
Felson et al.	(1)	[1986]	39	1-3 years	–	> 60
Hawley et al.	(2)	[1988]	75	1 year	Symptoms	were stable
Onghl et al.	(3)	[1990]	58	3.3 years	31	68
Mallison et al.	(4)	[1992]	28	2.2 years	–	61
Noregaard et al.	(5)	[1993]	83	4 years	10	71
Ledingham et al.	(6)	[1993]	72	4 years	26	74

ic issues. Only six of them (11,12,33,34,35,38) were conducted after 1990 and therefore used the American College of Rheumatology criteria for the classification of fibromyalgia. In the other trials, various sets of non-validated diagnostic criteria were utilized which often differed from one study to the other, thus making comparison across studies difficult.

Most studies evaluated a small number of patients [mean: 50 patients; median: 42 patients; range 11-208] and follow-up was short [mean: 8 weeks; median: 6 weeks; range 2-26 weeks]. The outcome measures differed widely among the trials with only a few defining a primary outcome that described clinically meaningful improvement (11,12,35). Five trials only incorporated functional outcome measures (11,19,23,30,35). Four of the 32 studies measured compliance (8,11,19,31) and the same number commented on co-intervention (11,21,29,32). Prognostic factors were evaluated in five studies (11,13,14,35,38). None of the trials has evaluated the overall cost of the interventions.

Taking into account the methodologic limitations in the design of the majority of these trials, the following conclusions can nevertheless be made: 1. Complete symptomatic remission is rarely, if ever, seen with any of the treatment modalities studied so far; 2. Anti-inflammatory medications, including corticosteroids and NSAID are generally ineffective; 3. Low-dose amitriptyline and cyclobenzaprine are the pharmacologic agents that have been the most extensively studied. In the short-term [one to three months], these drugs provide significant clinical improvement in 15 to 20 percent of patients, which is statistically higher than what is observed in patients receiving a placebo. However, the superiority of these drugs over placebo for longer periods of intake has yet to be demonstrated and will

TABLE 2. Randomized controlled clinical trials in fibromyalgia.

Reference	Treatment	n	evaluated	ACR criteria	Trial Duration	Type¶	Compliance	Co-interventions	Comments
Moldofsky [25]	Chlorpromazine Tryptophan	15	[15]	No	3 weeks	1	No	No	Chlorpromazine improved sleep and pain
Clarke [22]	Prednisone Placebo [PL]	20	[20]	No	2 weeks	2	No	No	Prednisone ineffective
Carette [7]	Amitriptyline [AM] Placebo	70	[59]	No	9 weeks	1	No	No	AM improved sleep, patient and physician global assess.
Goldenberg [8]	Amitriptyline Naprosyn Combination Placebo	52	[58]	No	6 weeks	1	Yes	No	AM improved pain, sleep, fatigue and myalgic scores. Naprosyn added little
Ferraccioli [37]	EMG-BFB Sham EMG-BFB	12	[12]	No	8 weeks	1	No	No	EMG-BFB improved pain, stiffness and tender points. Possible long-term benefit
McCain [31]§	CVR training FLEX training	42	[38]	No	20 weeks	1	Yes	No	CVR training improved fitness and pain threshold scores
Caruso [24]	Dothiepin Placebo	60	[52]	No	8 weeks	1	No	No	Dothiepin improved pain and tender points
Tavoni [20]	S-adenosyl-methionine [SAMe] Placebo	25	[17]	No	3 weeks	2	No	No	SAMe decreased the number of tender points and improved scores on the Hamilton Depression Scale
Bennett [13]	Cyclobenzaprine [CY]/Placebo	120	[120]	No	12 weeks	1	No	No	CY improved sleep, pain, muscle tightness and overall assessment
Yunus [18]	Ibuprofen Placebo	46	[43]	No	3 weeks	1	No	No	No difference between ibuprofen and placebo
Scudds [9]	Amitriptyline Placebo	39	[36]	No	4 weeks	2	No	No	AM improved pain, myalgic scores and pt global assessment

TABLE 2 (continued)

Reference	Treatment	n	evaluated	ACR criteria	Trial Duration	Type¶	Compliance	Co-interventions	Comments
Quimby [15]	Cyclobenzaprine Placebo	45	[40]	No	6 weeks	1	No	No	CY improved pain, sleep, stiffn. pt and phy overall assessments.
Hamaty [14]	Cyclobenzaprine Placebo	11	[7]	No	21 weeks	2	No	No	CY improved sleep but not pain
Fisher [36]	Homeopathic Placebo	30	[-]	No	4 weeks	2	No	No	Homeopathic treatment improved pain and decreased tender points
Caruso [26]	5-Hydroxy-Tryptophan [5HT] Placebo	50	[46]	No	4 weeks	1	No	No	5HT improved pain, stiffness, sleep fatigue and decreased tender points
Russell [19]	Alprazolan Ibuprofen Combination Placebo	78	[63]	No	6 weeks	1	Yes	No	No differences between the 4 groups except on post hoc analysis which favored comb.
Reynolds [16]	Cyclobenzaprine Placebo	12	[9]	No	4 weeks	2	No	No	CY improved sleep and evening fatigue
Jacobsen [21]	S-adenosyl-methionine Placebo	44	[38]	No	6 weeks	1	No	Yes	SAMe improved pain, fatigue, morning stiffness and mood
Jaeschke [10]	Amitriptyline Placebo	22	[22]	No	2 weeks	3	No	No	AM effective in 25% of patients as measured by questionnaire and count of tender points
Drewes [27]	Zopiclone Placebo	45	[41]	No	12 weeks	1	No	No	Zo improved sleep complaints and tiredness during the day.
Haanen [32]§	Hypnotherapy 8 hours/3month Physical training 1-2h/week	40	[37]	No	12 weeks	1	No	Yes	Hypnotherapy superior for pain, fatigue, sleep and patient global assessment. F/U for add. 3 months

Study	Intervention	n	Ref		Duration	Type			Results
Mengshoel [33]§	Physical training 2/week, No change in activities	35	[25]	Yes	20 weeks	1	No	No	Improved dynamic endurance work performance for the upper extremity in treated group.
Deluze (38)	Electroacupuncture [EA], Sham EA	70	[55]	Yes	3 weeks	1	No	No	EA improved pain, sleep, patient and physician global assessments
Pattrick [29]	Chlormezazone, Placebo	42	[41]	No	6 weeks	1	No	Yes	Chlormezazone comparable to placebo
Gronblad [28]	Zopiclone [Zo], Placebo	49	[33]	No	8 weeks	1	No	No	No difference between Zo and PL on any of the parameters studied
Santandrea [17]	Cyclobenzaprine 10 mg/day 30 mg/day	40	[?]	No	2 weeks	2	No	No	Both dosages effective but more side effects with 30 mg than 10 mg
Carette [11]	Amitriptyline Cyclobenzaprine Placebo	208	[184]	Yes	26 weeks	1	Yes	Yes	AM and CY effective at one month No diffrence between active drugs and placebo at 3 and 6 months
Burckhardt [35]§	Education [ED] ED+physical training Wait-list control	99	[86]	Yes	6 weeks	1	No	No	Self-efficacy improved in active groups
Wolfe * [30]	Somatostatin Placebo	82	[56]	?	3 weeks	1	–	–	Somatostatin comparable to placebo
Wolfe * [23]	Fluoxetine Placebo	42	[20]	?	6 weeks	1	–	–	Fluoxetine comparable to placebo
Martin * [34]§	CVR Exercise Relaxation	60	[38]	Yes	6 weeks	1	–	–	Aerobic exercise improve aerobic fitness and tender points
Carette * [12]	Amitriptyline Placebo	22	[22]	Yes	8 weeks	2	–	–	AM better than placebo

¶ Type: 1: parallel trial; 2: cross-over design; 3: N-of-1 design trial
§ These trials were not double-blind due to the nature of the intervention
* Abstracts

require studies with total enrollment of a minimum of 250-350 patients; 4. Patients with fibromyalgia can exercise and improve their cardiovascular fitness significantly without experiencing an exacerbation of their symptoms. However, the benefit of exercise in reducing the symptoms of pain and stiffness and in improving the quality of sleep appears to be marginal; 5. The data available for the other treatment modalities, including multidisciplinary treatment programs, are insufficient at this time to make specific recommendations; 6. Future studies on treatment modalities in fibromyalgia should include assessment of cost.

REFERENCES

1. Felson DT, Goldenberg DL: The natural history of fibromyalgia. Arthritis Rheum 29:1522-1526, 1986.

2. Hawley DJ, Wolfe F, Cathey MA: Pain, functional disability and psychological status: a 12 month study of severity in fibromyalgia. J Rheumatol 15: 1551-1556, 1988.

3. Ongchi DR, Dill ER, Katz RS: How often do fibromyalgia patients improve? Arthritis Rheum 33: S136, 1990.

4. Malleson PN, Al-Matar M, Petty RE: Idiopathic musculoskeletal pain syndromes in children. J Rheumatol 19:1786-1789, 1992.

5. Norregaard J, Bulow PM, Prescott E, Jacobsen S, Danneskiold-Samsoe: A four-year follow-up study in fibromyalgia. relationship to chronic fatigue syndrome. Scan J Rheumatol 22:35-38, 1993.

6. Ledingham J, Doherty S, Doherty M: Primary fibromyalgia syndrome: an outcome study. Br J Rheumatol 32: 139-142, 1993.

7. Carette S, McCain GA, Bell DA, Fam AG: Evaluation of amitriptyline in primary fibrositis: a double-blind, placebo-controlled study. Arthritis Rheum 29: 655-659, 1986.

8. Goldenberg DL, Felson DT, Dinerman H: A randomized, controlled trial of amitriptyline and naproxen in the treatment of patients with fibromyalgia. Arthritis Rheum 29: 1371-1377, 1986.

9. Scudds RA, McCain GA, Rollman GB, Harth M: Improvements in pain responsiveness in patients with fibrositis after successful treatment with amitriptyline. J Rheumatol [Suppl 19]: 98-103, 1989.

10. Jaeschke R, Adachi J, Guyatt G, Keller J, Wong B: Clinical usefulness of amitriptyline in fibromyalgia: the results of 23 N-of-1 randomized controlled trials. J Rheumatol 18: 447-451, 1991.

11. Carette S, Bell MJ, Reynolds WJ, Haraoui B, McCain GA, Bykerk VP, Edworthy SM, Baron M, Koehler BE, Fam AG, Bellamy N, Guimont C: Comparison of amitriptyline, cyclobenzaprine, and placebo in the treatment of fibromyalgia: a randomized, double-blind clinical trial. Arthritis Rheum 37: 32-40, 1994.

12. Carette S, Oakson G, Guimont C, Steriade M: Sleep electroencephalography [EEG] and the clinical response to amitriptyline in patients with fibromyalgia. Arthritis Rheum 36: S250, 1993.

13. Bennett RM, Gatter RA, Campbell SM, Andrews RP, Clark SR, Sarola JA: A comparison of cyclobenzaprine and placebo in the management of fibrositis: a double-blind controlled study. Arthritis Rheum 31: 1535- 1542, 1988.

14. Hamaty D, Valentine JL, Howard R, Howard CW, Wakefield V, Patten MS: The plasma endorphin, prostaglandin and catecholamine profile of patients with fibrositis treated with cyclobenzaprine and placebo: a 5-month study. J Rheumatol 16 [suppl 19]: 164-168, 1989.

15. Quimby LG, Gratwick GM, Whitney CD, Block SR: A randomized trial of cyclobenzaprine for the treatment of fibromyalgia. J Rheumatol 16 [suppl 19]: 140-143, 1989.

16. Reynolds WJ, Moldofsky H, Saskin P, Lue FA: The effects of cyclobenzaprine on sleep physiology and symptoms in patients with fibromyalgia. J Rheumatol 18: 452-454, 1991.

17. Santandrea S, Montrone F, Sarzi-Puttini P, Boccassini L, Caruso: A double-blind crossover study of two cyclobenzaprine regimens in primary fibromyalgia syndrome. J Int Med Res 21: 74-80, 1993.

18. Yunus MB, Masi AT, Aldag JC: Short term effects of ibuprofen in primary fibromyalgia syndrome: a double blind, placebo controlled trial. J Rheumatol 16: 527-532, 1989.

19. Russell IL, Flether EM, Michalek JE, McBroom PC, Hester GG: Treatment of primary fibrositis/fibromyalgia syndrome with ibuprofen and alprazolan: a double-blind, placebo-controlled study. Arthritis Rheum 34: 552-560, 1991.

20. Tavoni A, Vitali C, Bombardieri S, Pasero G: Evaluations of S- adenosylmethionine in primary fibromyalgia: a double-blind, crossover study. Am J Med [Suppl 5A] 83: 107-110, 1987.

21. Jacobsen S, Danneskiold-Samsoe B, Andersen RB: Oral S- adenosylmethionine in primary fibromyalgia. Double-blind clinical evaluation. Scan J Rheumatol 20: 294-302, 1991.

22. Clark S, Tindall E, Bennett RM: A double blind crossover trial of prednisone versus placebo in the treatment of fibrositis. J Rheumatol 12: 980-983, 1985.

23. Wolfe F, Cathey MA, Hawley DJ: A double-blind placebo controlled trial of fluoxetine in patients with fibromyalgia. Arthritis Rheum 36: S 220, 1993.

24. Caruso I, Sarzi Puttini PC, Boccassini L et al: Double-blind study of dothiepin versus placebo in the treatment of primary fibromyalgia syndrome. J Int Med Res 15: 154-159, 1987.

25. Moldofsky H, Lue FA: The relationship of alpha and delta EEG frequencies to pain and mood in "fibrositis" patients treated with chlorpromazine and L-tryptophan. Electroencephalogy Clin Neurophysiol 50:71-80, 1980.

26. Caruso I, Sarzi Puttini P, Cazzola M, Azzolini V: Double-blind study of 5-hydroxytryptophan versus placebo in the treatment of primary fibromyalgia syndrome. J Int Med Res 18: 201-209, 1990.

27. Drewes AM, Andreasen A, Jennum P, Nielsen KD: Zopiclone in the treatment of sleep abnormalities in fibromyalgia. Scan J Rheumatol 20: 288-293, 1991.

28. Gronblad M, Nykanen J, Konttinen Y, Jarvinen E, Helve T: Effect of zopiclone on sleep quality, morning stiffness, widespread tenderness and pain and general discomfort in primary fibromyalgia patients. A double-blind randomized trial. Clin Rheumatol 12: 186-91, 1993.

29. Pattrick M, Swannell A, Doherty M: Chlormezanone in primary fibromyalgia syndrome: a double blind placebo controlled study. Br J Rheumatol 32: 55-58, 1993.

30. Wolfe F, Mullis M, Cathey MA: A double-blind placebo controlled trial of somatostatin in fibromyalgia. Arthritis Rheum 34: S 188, 1991.

31. McCain GA, Bell DA, Mai FM, Halliday PE: A controlled study of the effects of a supervised cardiovascular fitness training program on the manifestations of primary fibromyalgia. Arthritis Rheum 31: 1135-1141, 1988.

32. Haanen HCM, Hoenderdos HTW, van Romunde LKJ, Hop WCJ, Mallee C, Terwiel JP, Hekster GB: Controlled trial of hypnotherapy in the treatment of refractory fibromyalgia. J Rheumatol 18: 72-75, 1991.

33. Mengshoel AM, Komnaes HB, Forre O: The effects of 20 weeks of physical fitness training in female patients with fibromyalgia. Clin Exp Rheumatol 10: 345-349, 1992.

34. Martin L, Edworthy SM, MaxIntosh B, Nutting A, Butterwick D, Cook J: Is exercise helpful in the treatment of fibromyalgia? Arthritis Rheum 36: S 251, 1993.

35. Burckhardt CS, Mannerkorpi K, Hedenberg L, Bjelle A: A randomized, controlled clinical trial of education and physical training for women with fibromyalgia. J Rheumatol 21: 714-720. 1994.

36. Fisher P, Greenwood A, Huskisson EC, Turner P, Belon P: Effect of homeopathic treatment on fibrositis [primary fibromyalgia]. BMJ 299: 365-366, 1989.

37. Ferraccioli G, Ghirelli L, Scita F, Nolli M, Mozzani M, Fontana S, Scorsonelli M, Tridenti A, DeRisio C: EMG-biofeedback training in fibromyalgia syndrome. J Rheumatol 14: 820-825, 1987.

38. Deluze C, Bosia L, Zirbs A, Chantraine A, Vischer: Electroacupuncture in fibromyalgia: results of a controlled trial. BMJ 305: 1249-1252, 1992.

Cognitive Behavior Therapy and the Treatment of Chronic Fatigue Syndrome

Michael Sharpe

WHAT IS CHRONIC FATIGUE SYNDROME?

The term chronic fatigue syndrome [CFS] has been proposed to describe a group of patients who complain of fatigue which is chronic [of at least six months duration], disabling, and associated with other symptoms including muscle pain and poor concentration, but unexplained by disease (1,2). The syndrome is unlikely to be homogenous and overlaps with others in which fatigue and pain are prominent symptoms. These include chronic pain syndromes, fibromyalgia, and anxiety and depressive disorders (3).

WHAT IS COGNITIVE BEHAVIOR THERAPY?

Cognitive behavior therapy [CBT] is a form of therapy and not a specific treatment. Its defining characteristic is an emphasis on the role of patients'

Dr. Michael Sharpe is Tutor in Psychiatry, University of Oxford in Oxford, UK.
Address correspondence to: Dr. Michael Sharpe, Warneford Hospital, Oxford OX3 7JX UK.

The author wishes to acknowledge his collaborators: Ms. Ann Hackmann, Dr. Keith Hawton, Ms. Ivana Klimes, Dr. T.E.A. Peto, Ms. Sue Simkin and Professor D. Warrell.
The Oxford trial was funded by the Wellcome Trust.

[Haworth co-indexing entry note]: "Cognitive Behavior Therapy and the Treatment of Chronic Fatigue Syndrome." Sharpe, Michael. Co-published simultaneously in the *Journal of Musculoskeletal Pain* (The Haworth Medical Press, an imprint of The Haworth Press, Inc.) Vol. 3, No. 2, 1995, pp. 141-147; and: *Fibromyalgia, Chronic Fatigue Syndrome, and Repetitive Strain Injury: Current Concepts in Diagnosis, Management, Disability, and Health Economics* (ed: Andrew Chalmers et al.) The Haworth Medical Press, an imprint of The Haworth Press, Inc., 1995, pp. 141-147. Multiple copies of this article/chapter may be purchased from The Haworth Document Delivery Center [1-800-3-HAWORTH; 9:00 a.m. - 5:00 p.m. (EST)].

© 1995 by The Haworth Press, Inc. All rights reserved.

thoughts, basic beliefs [cognitions] and behavior in perpetuating distress, symptoms and disability. The principal aim of therapy is to help patients to reevaluate and, if necessary, change the way they think about and cope with a problem with the aim of improving their well-being. CBT may be used as an individual therapy, or as a group therapy; it may focus primarily on the patient's cognitions or on their behavior; it may simply aim to achieve a better adjustment to a problem or to help the patient overcome it.

Although initially developed as a treatment for depression (4), CBT is now also widely used in the treatment of anxiety, phobias, panic and eating disorders. More recently, CBT has been adapted for use in the treatment of patients with predominantly somatic complaints unexplained by organic disease. It has already been shown to be of value in the treatment of patients with atypical chest pain, back pain, headache, irritable bowel syndrome, and hypochondriasis (5).

COGNITIVE BEHAVIOR THERAPY
AND CHRONIC FATIGUE SYNDROME

Why use CBT for patients with CFS? There is, at present, no accepted therapy for patients with CFS. The case for adding CBT to the list of possible treatments for CFS can be made on both pragmatic and on theoretical grounds. Pragmatically, CBT may considered to be of benefit in improving emotional and behavioral adjustment to CFS whatever the basic cause of the symptoms. Theoretically, CBT may be seen to follow from a cognitive behavioral theory of the etiology of CFS.

A cognitive behavioral theory of CFS. Patients with CFS have high rates of depression and anxiety, tend to believe in physical disease as an explanation for their symptoms and to cope with their illness by avoiding activity (6,7). Furthermore, patients who have a strong belief in disease have a poorer outcome (8). Theoretical models that aim to explain the perpetuation of symptoms and disability in patients with CFS in terms of cognitive, behavioral and emotional factors have been proposed (9,10). The symptoms of fatigue and muscle pain may result from a variety of factors including depression, anxiety and inactivity. If these are attributed by the patient to physical disease, any activity that exacerbates the symptoms may be avoided for fear of "exacerbating the disease." The consequent anxiety, depression, frustration and inactivity tend to perpetuate the symptoms. Consequently, the patient becomes trapped in a vicious circle [see Figure 1].

FIGURE 1. A cognitive behavioral model of illness perpetuation in CFS.

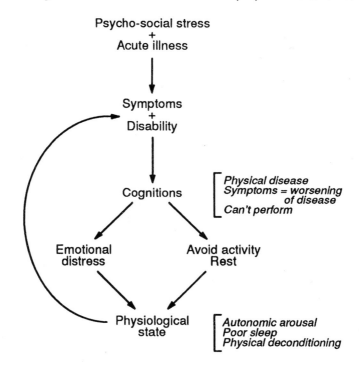

HOW EFFECTIVE IS CBT IN THE TREATMENT OF CFS?

The validity of the cognitive behavioral model remains to be established. Several centers are already treating patients with CFS using a cognitive behavioral approach however, and three published studies have formally evaluated various forms of CBT in patients with CFS. We are also conducting a controlled trial of CBT for patients with CFS in Oxford.

The National Hospital study. The first study was an uncontrolled case series of outpatients and patients at the National Hospital For Nervous Diseases in London (7). The form of CBT employed in this study was individual therapy focused on a gradual increase of activity with the aim of overcoming avoidance. Treatment was by a nurse therapist over a number of months. Patients who were depressed were also given an antidepressant drug. Fifty severely disabled patients meeting criteria for CFS (2) were offered treatment but eighteen refused. Of the 32 patients treated, there was a clinically significant improvement in symptoms and in functioning for 22/32 [69%], which was maintained at 3 months follow-up. However, 5 patients dropped out before treatment was completed.

The refusal and dropout rate in this study was too high to permit an evaluation of the effectiveness of the therapy. Furthermore, the use of combined pharmacological and non-pharmacological treatment, and the uncontrolled design of the study, complicate interpretation of the results. Nonetheless, this study indicated that something could be done for patients with CFS, and highlighted the potential role of CBT.

The New York study. This study was a *non-randomized* controlled study of CBT given as a group therapy for 22 patients with CFS (11). The aim of the therapy was to improve the patients adjustment to illness by challenging negative thinking and encouraging acceptance of a limitation on activity. The patients met criteria for CFS (1) and almost half also met criteria for major depressive disorder. Treatment was given over 6 to 9 weeks. At the end of treatment the CBT treated group were not significantly different from an untreated comparison group of treatment refusers on measures of fatigue and other symptoms. Further analysis of the results suggested that a higher depression scores at baseline predicted a positive response to treatment.

The negative result of this non-randomized trial is difficult to interpret. However, the cognitive behavioral model would predict that a treatment that did not challenge the patients' belief in a physical disease or aimed to overcome behavioral avoidance would be unlikely to produce significant change, although the observed reduction in self-critical cognitions might be expected to reduce depression.

The Prince Henry Hospital study. This study from Sydney, Australia is the only randomized controlled trial of CBT for CFS. It compared a form of CBT with standard medical management (12). The form of CBT used was similar to that employed in the National Hospital Study in that it included an emphasis on graded increases in activity. However, the patients' beliefs that they had a physical disease was not specifically challenged and the therapy was relatively brief [6 bi-weekly sessions of less than one hour].

Sixty-eight patients were recruited with a mean illness duration of over 5 years. None either refused CBT, or dropped out from this treatment. There was, however, no significant difference between the groups in the measures of distress or disability at the end of treatment or after a 7-month follow-up period, with both groups of patients reporting a reduction in fatigue and depression over the follow-up period. One might conclude from this study that this brief form of CBT is no more effective than careful medical follow-up in patients with CFS of long duration.

The Oxford study. Thus, the only study to date suggesting that CBT is effective in reducing fatigue and disability in patients with CFS was the National Hospital study which employed intensive individual therapy aimed at producing behavioral change and challenging the patient's attribution of symptoms to organic disease. The fact that subsequent trials have not challenged the patients' attributions might explain both their greater acceptability to patients and their relative ineffectiveness.

In Oxford, we have recently completed a randomized controlled trial of intensive CBT for patients with CFS (13). This trial aimed to avoid the limitations of previous studies. The CBT was intensive and comprised 16 one-hour individual treatment sessions over 4 months. Considerable attention was paid to the negotiation of a formulation of the illness that was acceptable to both patient and therapist and which formed the basis of a collaborative approach. The treatment aimed to overcome patients' avoidance of activity and to help them re-evaluate the accuracy and helpfulness of their attribution of symptoms to organic disease. Where necessary, it also addressed patients' unrealistic expectations of themselves, and self-critical thinking, and included problem-solving techniques for social difficulties. The components of the therapy are listed in Table 1.

Sixty consecutive referrals who met criteria for CFS (2) and who had been ill for less than 10 years were recruited from an infectious disease outpatient clinic. CBT was compared with standard medical care by hospital and primary care physician. Outcome was measured at one, three and eight months after the end of therapy and included both assessments of

TABLE 1. Components of the cognitive behavioral therapy of CBT [Oxford trial].

1. **Engagement**	Establishing collaborative approach Producing individual formulation
2. **Behavioral change**	Increasing activity Overcoming avoidance

3. **Cognitive change**
    A. Illness
    B. Standards
	
	Re-evaluation of disease attribution
	Reduction in concern about symptoms
	Reappraisal of excessive standards
	Re-evaluation of self-critical attitudes

4. **Problems solving**	Social and occupational difficulties Implications of recovery

overall state by an independent assessor, and patient-rated measures of functional impairment and of symptoms.

Two patients refused randomization. None dropped out of treatment. Treatment was often difficult, however. Some patients were reluctant to accept a treatment that directly addressed psychological factors; other persons sometimes reinforced the patients' existing beliefs and discouraged them from increasing their activity level; some patients were receiving financial benefits that they would loose if they were seen to improve; some did not wish to return to work until they had changed their career direction. Despite these difficulties substantial gains were made. The question of whether these gains were significantly greater with CBT than with standard medical care must await final analysis of the results.

CONCLUSION

The evaluation of CBT in the treatment of CFS is justified on both pragmatic and theoretical grounds. With the exception of the first reported case series, treatment trials have been disappointing. This lack of efficacy may reflect the use of weak and theoretically sub-optimal forms of CBT. A recent study from Oxford has achieved excellent patient compliance despite challenging patients beliefs about their illness. The final judgement of the role of CBT in CFS must await the result of this and other studies currently in progress. Future cognitive behavioral approaches will require further refinement in the challenging of patients' illness beliefs and effective ways of overcoming social and interpersonal factors that tend to perpetuate illness.

REFERENCES

1. Schluederberg A, Straus SE, Peterson PK, Blumenthal S, Komaroff AL, Spring SB, Landay AL, Buchwald D: Chronic Fatigue Syndrome Research: definition and medical outcome. Ann Intern Med 1992;117:325-31.

2. Sharpe MC, Archard LC, Banatvala JE, Borysiewicz LK, Clare AW, David AS, et al: A report-chronic fatigue syndrome: guidelines for research. J R Soc Med 1991;84:118-21.

3. Sharpe MC. Fatigue and chronic fatigue syndrome. Curr Opin Psychiatry 1992;5:207-12.

4. Beck AT; Rush AJ; Shaw BF, et al: Cognitive therapy of depression. New York: Guilford Press; 1979.

5. Sharpe MC, Peveler R, Mayou R: The psychological treatment of patients with functional somatic symptoms: a practical guide. J Psychosom Res 1992; 36:515-29.

6. Sharpe MC, Hawton KE, Seagraott V, Pasvol G: Patients who present with fatigue: a follow up of referrals to an infectious diseases clinic. BMJ 1992; 305:147-52.

7. Butler S, Chalder T, Ron M, Wessely S: Cognitive behavior therapy in chronic fatigue syndrome. J Neurol Neurosurg Psychiatry 1991;54:153-8.

8. Wilson A, Hickie I, Lloyd A, Hadzi-Pavlovic D, Boughton C, Dwyer J, Wakefield D: Longitudinal study of outcome of chronic fatigue syndrome. BMJ 1994;308:756-9.

9. Wessely S, David AS, Butler S, Chalder T: Management of chronic (postviral) fatigue syndrome. J R Coll Gen Pract 1989;39:26-9.

10. Sharpe MC: Psychiatric management of PVFS. Br Med Bull 1991; 47:989-1006.

11. Friedberg F, Krupp LB: A comparison of cognitive behavioral treatment for Chronic Fatigue Syndrome and primary depression. Clin Infect Dis 1994;18 (supplement 1):s105-9.

12. Lloyd AR, Hickie I, Brockman A, Hickie C, Wilson A, Dwyer J, Wakefield D: Immunologic and psychologic therapy for patients with chronic fatigue syndrome: a double-blind, placebo-controlled trial. Am J Med 1993;94:197-203.

13. Sharpe MC: Non-pharmacological appraoches to treatment: Chronic Fatigue Syndrome, CIBA Foundation Symposium 173. Edited by GR Brock, J Whelan, John Wiley & Sons, Toronto, 1993, pp. 298-317.

Evaluation of Myofascial Pain and Dysfunction Syndromes and Their Response to Low Level Laser Therapy

Pekka J. Pöntinen
Olavi Airaksinen

SUMMARY. Objectives: The purpose of this article is to present a method for evaluation and follow-up of myofascial pain and dysfunction syndromes [MPS].

Findings: Since 1987, our study group has tested various pressure threshold [PTH] and tolerance [PTO] meters. Reliability and validity studies have confirmed their place as a semiobjective estimate of MPS. PTH measurement facilitates exact location of trigger regions and tender spots. PTO reveals abnormal sensitivity to pain. Tissue compliance [TCO] measurement provides an objective method to evaluate muscle spasms and tension. A trial treatment with low-energy laser directed to trigger points [TPs] may elevate PTH and maximal grasping force [MGF] instantaneously and thus con-

Pekka J. Pöntinen, MD, PhD, is Associate Professor, Institute of Clinical Sciences, Department of Neurology, Tampere University and Associate Professor, Department of Physiology, Kuopio University, Finland.

Olavi Airaksinen, MD, PhD, is Associate Professor and Clinical Director, Department of Physical Medicine and Rehabilitation, Kuopio University Hospital, Finland.

Address correspondence to: Pekka J. Pöntinen, MD, PhD, Pikkusaarenkuja 4 B 77, FIN-33410 Tampere, Finland.

[Haworth co-indexing entry note]: "Evaluation of Myofascial Pain and Dysfunction Syndromes and Their Response to Low Level Laser Therapy." Pöntinen, Pekka J., and Olavi Airaksinen. Co-published simultaneously in the *Journal of Musculoskeletal Pain* (The Haworth Medical Press, an imprint of The Haworth Press, Inc.) Vol. 3, No. 2, 1995, pp. 149-154; and: *Fibromyalgia, Chronic Fatigue Syndrome, and Repetitive Strain Injury: Current Concepts in Diagnosis, Management, Disability, and Health Economics* (ed: Andrew Chalmers et al.) The Haworth Medical Press, an imprint of The Haworth Press, Inc., 1995, pp. 149-154. Multiple copies of this article/chapter may be purchased from The Haworth Document Delivery Center [1-800-3-HAWORTH; 9:00 a.m. - 5:00 p.m. (EST)].

© 1995 by The Haworth Press, Inc. All rights reserved.

firm the functional nature of a patient's disability. Surface electromyography and thermography reflect abnormalities in neuromuscular function and sympathetic activity and complete the evaluation.

Conclusions: Extended functional analysis, complemented with provocation and simple loading tests, provides a reliable and valid method for evaluation and follow-up of MPS patients.

KEYWORDS. Myofascial pain syndrome, pressure algometry, surface EMG, laser therapy, pain threshold

INTRODUCTION

Pain is a common denominator in myofascial pain syndrome [MPS]. Pain scales, visual analogue scales, pain questionnaires, pain drawings and personality profiles can only reflect subjective, emotionally loaded facets of pain behavior. In the normal clinical situation, it is impossible to follow changes of central pain modulating substances. Other practical measures are needed.

Since 1987, our study group has tested various pressure threshold [PTH] and pressure tolerance [PTO] meters. Reliability and validity studies have confirmed their place as a semiobjective estimate of MPS (1-4). PTH measurement facilitates exact location of the most hyperalgesic points and regions in muscles and soft tissue (3). PTO examines sensitivity to pain which may reflect psychological mechanisms (3). Tissue compliance [TCO] measurement provides an objective method to evaluate muscle tightness and tension for diagnostic purposes and follow-up studies (5). Muscle fatigue is a typical sign in MPS (6). A simple hand dynamometer for grasping force measurement is a useful tool to estimate muscle force and endurance. EMG and thermography reflect changes and abnormalities in neuromuscular function and sympathetic activity (7-9). Using these techniques our aim has been to create a simple and reliable method for the functional analysis of MPS and PFM.

METHODS

Algometry

Specially adapted pressure-gauges are available to measure tissue sensitivity to pressure. These instruments enable clinicians and researchers to accurately detect tender points, and trigger points [TPs], and to measure the patient's PTH and PTO. They allow the clinician/researcher to objectively compare the sensitivity of active and passive [latent] TPs and to monitor the response to therapy. TCO reflects many variables, such as rigidity, spasticity or edema, for instance, in an area. The more rigid an area, the shallower the depth of penetration of a blunt probe applied with predetermined pressure.

1. PTH is routinely measured with a PTH-meter [Pain Diagnostics & Thermography Inc., 233 East Shore Rd, Suite 108, Great Neck, NY 11023] consisting of a pressure gauge with a plunger ending to a rubber disk with a surface of 1 cm^2. The gauge is calibrated in kg/cm^2 with a range of 0-11 kg/cm^2. Pressure is applied in a straight angle to a defined surface of the body through the rubber disk. The patient is asked to mark the first pain sensation either verbally or with a hand sign while increasing the pressure at the speed of about 1 kg/cm^2/s. MPS patients and patients with PFM have an abnormally low PTH. Their muscles often react with a muscle twitch or contraction when the applied pressure exceeds the PTH. This is a more reliable sign than any verbal announcement. To obtain reliable data the measurement should be repeated.

In healthy subjects, mean normal values for PTH are 5.4-9.0 kg/cm^2 in males and 3.7-6.8 kg/cm^2 in females (1-3). Significant differences include the following: the lumbar paravertebral mm., both lateral and medial, mm. glutei and to a lesser degree the deltoid and infraspinatus muscles were distinguished by a higher PTH than the other muscles tested, according to Fischer (3). Active trigger points may react to pressures as low as 0.5-1.5 kg/cm^2. These values may increase 3- to 6-fold after a successful TP therapy.

2. PTO measurement. A PTO-meter is similar to a PTH-meter, but the range of the pressure gauge is 0-17 kg/cm^2 for practical reasons. PTO-measurement should be done over a normal muscle [e.g., m. deltoideus] and bone or periost [lower medial tibia/shin bone] exploring non-tender areas and avoiding tender ones. The pressure is increased beyond the PTH until pain sensation becomes unbearable–to the person's tolerance. It is important to know both muscle and bone tolerance levels for diagnostic and prognostic purposes. Patients having abnormally low muscle and bone tolerance are not suitable for any stimulation or manipulative therapy before their PTO returns to normal level. Instead of analgesics or physical therapy they may need antidepressants and biofeedback or psychotherapy. Low muscle PTO is seen in PMF, hypothyroidism and with estrogen deficiency. Normally, there should be a clear margin between PTH and PTO values.

3. Tissue compliance [TCO] measurement. A TCO-meter is a hand-held instrument with a pressure gauge, similar to PTH- and PTO-meters, connected to a long shaft ending in a rubber disk [1 cm^2]. This shaft is pressed through a sliding disk into the tissue under examination. Compliance is expressed in mm of the depth of penetration and related to the force employed. Sequential measurement of gradually increasing preselected pressures [usually 1, 2, 3 and 4 kg/cm^2] allows construction of a TCO curve. Tissue compliance measurement documents muscle tone and its alterations in pathological conditions. It can be used to reveal muscle spasm, spasticity, rigidity as signs of augmented muscle tone or flaccidity as an early sign of dysfunctioning monosynaptic reflex arc (5).

Functional Analysis

1. Range of movement is the normal basis for joint and muscle evaluation. In MPS and PFM, muscle tension is abnormally high throughout the body. Therefore, a simple test, e.g., maximal incisival opening, may reflect the state of the whole body.

2. A simple hand dynamometer [Vigorimeter, Gebrüder Martin, Tutlingen, Germany] gives us useful information of the functional state of muscles. As fatigue or poor endurance is typical of MPS and PFM, the maximal grasping force [MGF] test should be repeated in a series of 10 measurements. A greater than 10% decrease in the MGF after 10 compressions is a sign of abnormal fatigue.

3. Endurance test. The subjects are asked to sit with the arms abducted 90 degrees as long as they can. Without MPS in the shoulder girdle or PFM, 4 minutes should be easily exceeded.

4. Trial of treatment. In MPS, laser therapy and, to a lesser extent, TENS, elevate PTH and MGF almost instantaneously when directed to relevant trigger points or regions and can be used to differentiate between peripheral and central mechanisms of pain and disability (10). To confirm the functional importance of the detected reactive TPs or regions an analgesic laser irradiation dose is given [1-2 J/TP; appr. 75-150 J/cm^2] and the functional analysis, including PTH and MGF, repeated. Restoration of normal or near-normal function confirms the role of trigger mechanism. If there is no change in 1-2 minutes a small laser irradiation dose [0.1-0.2 J/point] is given to the corresponding paravertebral tender site[s] inside the same segment. The immediate restoration of muscle strength confirms the segmental level in functional disorders.

5. Thermography [TG], liquid crystal or emission type, reflects changes in the sympathetic activity and peripheral circulation. TG can document hyperactive TPs as "hot spots" while the referred pain zone may show

either increased or decreased thermal emission. Although TG cannot be used alone as a diagnostic tool it may provide valuable information for early detection of reflex sympathetic dystrophy and allows for follow-up studies.

6. Surface electromyography [EMG] is used for documentation of abnormal muscular activity and reflects the fatigue phenomenon characteristic for MPS and PFM. This method has been applied to distinguish patients with musculoskeletal disorders from normals and to verify the reason for postoperative failed back syndrome (8). Abnormal muscle fatigue [poor endurance] is clearly demonstrated in loading tests under EMG-monitoring (9).

Provocation Tests

Many myofascial pain patients have so-called non-cardiac chest pain and hyperalgesia in their chest wall (11). Chest pain may be experienced during or just after physical or mental stress. Therefore, it is advisable to perform simple provocation tests to check patients' physiological reaction to stress. A simple static compression of a Vigorimeter ball with 1/3 of the MGF or weight bearing in the straight hand [1.0 kg for women, 1.5 kg for men] for 4 minutes may induce maximal loading on the left heart, and a corresponding elevation in diastolic and systolic pressures comparable to those during maximal isokinetic and dynamic exercise. Diastolic blood pressure exceeding 100 mmHg may be indicative of future hypertension in normotensive subjects.

RESULTS AND DISCUSSION

Repeated measurements during the course of treatment provide data for follow-up and correlate well with VAS and pain questionnaires. E.g., in a series of 54 MPS patients given low level laser therapy [IR 820 nm] to TPs PTH increased from 2.94 ± 1.44 to 6.56 ± 0.96 kg/cm^2 [P < 0.001] and MGF from 0.60 ± 0.28 to 1.03 ± 0.29 bar [P < 0.05], whereas VAS decreased from 44.6 ± 11.3 to 9.3 ± 6.4 [P < 0.001]. The effect was greater on the side with the initially lower PTH and MGF values.

For documentation and evaluation of MPS patients and their follow-up a battery of simple, easy-to-apply, and reliable tests and measurements is suggested. No single method alone can adequately show functional changes or pain relief.

REFERENCES

1. Airaksinen O, Pöntinen PJ: The reliability of the pain threshold algometry on latent myofascial trigger points in healthy Finnish students. 1st International Symposium on Myofascial Pain and Fibromyalgia, Minneapolis, Minn., 8-10 May 1989.

2. Pöntinen PJ, Vuoto L: Pressure algometry in low back pain patients and healthy controls. Myopain'92, 2nd World Congress on Myofascial Pain and Fibromyalgia, Copenhagen 17-20 August 1992.

3. Fischer AA: Application of pressure algometry in manual medicine. J Manual Medicine 5:145-150, 1990.

4. Hong C-Z, Chen Y-C, Pon CH, Yu J: Immediate effects of various physical medicine modalities on pain threshold of an active myofascial trigger point. J Musculoske Pain 1(2): 37-53, 1993.

5. Fischer AA: Tissue compliance meter for objective, quantitative documentation of soft tissue consistency and pathology. Arch Phys Med Rehabil 68: 122-125, 1987.

6. Jacobsen S, Danneskiold-Samsoe B: Dynamic muscular endurance in primary fibromyalgia compared with chronic myofascial pain syndrome. Arch Phys Med Rehabil 73: 170-173, 1992.

7. AMA Council Report: Thermography in neurological and musculoskeletal conditions. Thermology 2:600-607, 1987.

8. Sihvonen T, Herno A, Paljärvi L, Airaksinen O, Partanen J, Tapaninaho A: Local denervation atrophy of paraspinal muscles in postoperative failed back syndrome. Spine 18:575-581, 1993.

9. Kaljumäe U, Airaksinen O, Hänninen O: Knee extensor strength and relative fatigability after bicycle ergometer training. Arch Phys Med Rehabil (in press).

10. Pöntinen PJ: Technique of LLLT. Myofascial trigger points. In the book: Low Level Laser Therapy as a Medical Treatment Modality. Art Urpo Ltd, Tampere, 1992, pp. 56-79.

11. Wise CM, Semple EL, Dalton CB: Musculoskeletal chest wall syndromes in patients with noncardiac chest pain: a study of 100 patients. Arch Phys Med Rehabil 73:147-149, 1992.

Prognostic Indicators of Disability After a Work-Related Musculoskeletal Injury

Joan Crook
Harvey Moldofsky

SUMMARY. Objective: The aim of the study was to determine specific clinical and behavioral factors that prognostically influence return to work following a musculoskeletal work related injury.

Methods: A longitudinal cohort study was conducted on 148 randomly selected workers who had not returned to work in 3 months following musculoskeletal strain or sprain injury. The workers were interviewed at 3, 9, 15 and 21 months after injury. The WHO Classification of Impairment, Disabilities and Handicap was used as the conceptual framework. The analysis employed the Cox Proportional Hazards Regression model with allowance for time-dependent covariates.

Results: The relative rate of return to work for males was one-and-a-half times that for females and 20% less for every 10-year in-

Joan Crook, RN, PhD, is Professor, School of Nursing, Faculty of Health Sciences, McMaster University, Hamilton, Ontario, Canada.

Harvey Moldofsky, MD, is Professor of Psychiatry and Medicine, University of Toronto and Director, Center for Sleep and Chronobiology, Toronto, Ontario, Canada.

Address correspondence to: Joan Crook, RN, PhD, McMaster University, Faculty of Health Sciences, Room 3N28, 1200 Main Street West, Hamilton, Ontario, Canada L8N 3Z5.

Research supported by a grant from the Worker's Compensation Board of Ontario and the Ontario Workers' Compensation Institute.

[Haworth co-indexing entry note]: "Prognostic Indicators of Disability After a Work-Related Musculoskeletal Injury." Crook, Joan, and Harvey Moldofsky. Co-published simultaneously in the *Journal of Musculoskeletal Pain* (The Haworth Medical Press, an imprint of The Haworth Press, Inc.) Vol. 3, No. 2, 1995, pp. 155-159; and: *Fibromyalgia, Chronic Fatigue Syndrome, and Repetitive Strain Injury: Current Concepts in Diagnosis, Management, Disability, and Health Economics* (ed: Andrew Chalmers et al.) The Haworth Medical Press, an imprint of The Haworth Press, Inc., 1995, pp. 155-159. Multiple copies of this article/chapter may be purchased from The Haworth Document Delivery Center [1-800-3-HAWORTH; 9:00 a.m. - 5:00 p.m. (EST)].

© 1995 by The Haworth Press, Inc. All rights reserved.

crease in age. After controlling for gender and age, psychologic distress and functional disability were negatively associated with the rate of return to work. Psychologic distress associated with symptoms of fibromyalgia was prognostically important in the failure to return to work. Additionally, there was two times the rate of return to work for workers who were provided with light jobs.

Conclusions: These prognostic indicators require consideration for rehabilitation programs for workers who suffer musculoskeletal soft tissue injuries.

KEYWORDS. Prognosis, work disability, injured workers, musculoskeletal pain

INTRODUCTION

Musculoskeletal injuries pose a formidable health care problem for industry. Annually, 2% of the national force incurs industrially-related back injuries with approximately 1.4% of these injuries resulting in a period of work absence (1). Many people never seek medical care nor have any significant long-term disability. Despite the good prognosis for most episodes, musculoskeletal injuries consume considerable resources in medical care, absence from work and compensation benefits. Several studies have independently confirmed that it is the small number of chronic claimants who accrue most of the back injury costs (1,2,3). Little is known about those workers who are at a high risk for continued work disability. In addition, studies have shown that approximately 50% of patients with fibromyalgia report the onset of their non-restorative sleep, diffuse musculoskeletal pain, fatigue and psychological distress following a traumatic event (4). Because such traumatic events may occur at work, we hypothesized that workers who develop such a constellation of symptoms following a soft-tissue injury would encounter difficulty in returning to work.

It has become apparent that work disability is not a function of impairment and functional disability alone but depends on the interplay of various other factors. Occupational handicap may result from the demands of the job, the options available to the employer, and the range of personal, familial, rehabilitative and vocational options open to the individual (5).

The WHO Classification of Impairment, Disabilities and Handicaps (6) was used as the conceptual framework. The conceptual model underlying the ICIDH postulates a series of events consequent on an injury. The injury may give rise to impairments. Impairments are defined as temporary or permanent loss or abnormalities in the structure or functioning of the body and refer to symptoms. An impairment may give rise to disability. Disability is defined as a restriction or lack of ability to perform an activity in the manner or within the range considered normal. Impairment and disability may then lead to handicap. Handicap represents the end result of the consequences of the injury for the worker, and is partially determined by the social and cultural context. Handicap is defined as a disadvantage for a given individual that limits or prevents the fulfillment of a role that is considered normal for that individual.

The relationship between these planes of experience is not linear. Some of the factors that potentially mediate between impairment, disability and handicap after a work related injury, include the type of occupation, including the nature and heaviness of the work, the physical environment of the workplace, the social situation of the worker, and the resources available to the worker in dealing with the consequences of impairment or disability.

METHODS

The design of the study was a prospective longitudinal design of a randomly selected cohort of workers [N = 148] who had sustained a musculoskeletal soft tissue injury at work and had not returned to work by 3 months after injury. The sample was obtained from the files of the Workers Compensation Board of Ontario, Canada. The workers were interviewed and assessed at 3, 9, 15 and 21 months after injury. The workers were assessed with measures of pain [McGill Pain Questionnaire, visual analogue scale, University of Alabama Pain Behavior Scale (7), pain threshold tenderness with a dolorimeter, and number of body pain sites], fatigue (8), sleep complaint questionnaire, psychologic distress [SCL-90 questionnaire] (9) functional and social disabilities and handicaps.

RESULTS

The Study Group

There were slightly more males then females in the study group. The average age of the injured workers was 41 years. Male workers were more likely to be employed in manufacturing, trades, construction and the performance of laboring tasks than females. Female workers were more likely employed in the service, clerical and technical sectors. Most workers reported their accident to be the result of a strain or a fall. Sixty percent of the workers received immediate medical attention, half of whom were taken to the emergency room. Only two workers were admitted to a hospital.

Analysis

Several variables at the three-month assessment on enrollment into the study demonstrated a significant association with a decreased rate of returning to work: the relative rate of return to work for females was one third than for males, and 20% less for every 10-year increase in age. Functional disability and the psychological distress associated with symptoms were significantly and negatively associated with the rate of returning to work. The most functionally disabled workers were one-and-a-quarter times less likely to return to work [range 0-38]. The difference between those who scored lowest and highest [range 0-4] on the positive symptom distress scale (9) suggested that the most psychologically distressed workers were one-and-a-half times less likely to return to work.

A Cox Proportional model was developed to examine the prognostic importance of the symptoms associated with fibromyalgia in explaining work disability. The candidate variables that were entered into the model after controlling for the effects of age and gender were the number of pain sites, pain tenderness, sleep disturbance, fatigue and positive symptom distress. Positive symptom distress was significantly and negatively associated with the rate of returning to work. This result suggests that it is not the symptoms per se but the emotional distress associated with the symptoms that is most prognostically important in explaining work disability.

The Time Dependent Cox models that considered the clinical variables at each assessment period [3, 9, 15 and 21 months], identified physical independence handicap and functional disability to be negatively associated with return to work rates. Additionally, the employers' provision of a less physically demanding job or shorter work hours was positively associated with return to work rates. The relative rate of returning to work was two times more when the employees had a "light job" to which to return.

CONCLUSIONS

The significance of the research lies partly in the identification of disability and affective changes that occur over time that may signal the increasing vulnerability and potential for continued work disability. These prognostic indicators require consideration for rehabilitation programs for workers who suffer musculoskeletal soft tissue injury.

REFERENCES

1. Spitzer W (Chair) and Task Force: Report on the Quebec task force on spinal disorders. Spine (Suppl) 12: 75, 1987.

2. Webster BS, Snook SH: The cost of compensable low back pain. Journal of Occupational Medicine 32: 13-15, 1990.

3. Volinn E, Lai D, McKinney S, Loeser JD: When back pain becomes disabling: A regional analysis. Pain 33: 33-39, 1988.

4. Goldenberg DL: Do infections trigger fibromyalgia? Arthritis and Rheumatology 36: 1489-1492, 1993.

5. Yelin EH, Henke CJ, Epstein WV: Work disability among persons with musculoskeletal conditions. Arthritis and Rheumatism 29: 1322-1333, 1986.

6. World Health Organization: International classification of impairments, disabilities and handicaps. Geneva WHO.

7. Richards JS, Nepomuceno C, Riles M, Suer Z: Assessing pain behavior: The UAB pain behavior scale. Pain 14: 393-398, 1982.

8. Yoshitake H: Three characteristic patterns of subjective fatigue symptoms. Ergonomics 21: 231-233, 1978.

9. Derogatis LR: The SCL 90-R Clinical Psychometric Research. Baltimore, 1975.

Disability–
A Medical-Legal Concept;
The Physician's Role

George E. Ehrlich

SUMMARY. Objectives: The medical definitions of impairment [lesion, disability, the functional consequence thereof], and handicap [the social consequence, sanctified by the World Health Organization], differ from the legal concepts, in which impairment encompasses some of disability, while disability encompasses most of handicap. The medical testimony provides evidence; the designated legal representative [judge, arbitrator or panel] determines whether disability is present, its extent, and the likely duration, based on the medical evidence and other factors. This brief personal review addresses some of the shadings and conflicts the encounter between two disciplines produces.

Findings: Contradictions in "science" are adjudged on the preponderance of evidence, often an exercise in biostatistics, and the law representative sometimes makes medical judgments, whilst physicians and other health care professionals, because of training and humanitarian aims, often create the very dilemma they want to forestall. In relating the impairment to a temporally antecedent event, to permit a decision of casual or causal, Berkson's fallacy comes into play.

George E. Ehrlich, MO, FACP, MACR, is Adjunct Professor of Medicine, University of Pennsylvania School of Medicine and Adjunct Professor of Clinical Medicine, New York University School of Medicine.

Address correspondence to: George E. Ehrlich, MD, One Independence Place 1101, 241 South Sixth Street, Philadelphia, PA 19106-3731.

[Haworth co-indexing entry note]: "Disability–A Medical-Legal Concept; The Physician's Role." Ehrlich, George E. Co-published simultaneously in the *Journal of Musculoskeletal Pain* (The Haworth Medical Press, an imprint of The Haworth Press, Inc.) Vol. 3, No. 2, 1995, pp. 161-168; and: *Fibromyalgia, Chronic Fatigue Syndrome, and Repetitive Strain Injury: Current Concepts in Diagnosis, Management, Disability, and Health Economics* (ed: Andrew Chalmers et al.) The Haworth Medcial Press, an imprint of The Haworth Press, Inc., 1995, pp. 161-168. Multiple copies of this article/chapter may be purchased from The Haworth Document Delivery Center [1-800-3-HAWORTH; 9:00 a.m. - 5:00 p.m. (EST)].

© 1995 by The Haworth Press, Inc. All rights reserved.

161

Conclusions: The World Health Organization sequence, breaking down the problem into its various components, permits the physician to appreciate the evidentiary portions of the problem and thus to define disability medically in such a way that the "safety net" works appropriately.

KEYWORDS. Disability, impairment, medical testimony, prognosis, medicolegal controversies

A pox of this gout! or, a gout of this pox! for the one or the other plays the rogue with my great toe.

Falstaff...

It is no great matter if I do halt; I shall have the wars for my color, and my pensions shall seem the more reasonable. A good wit will make use of anything. I will turn the diseases to commodity.

Henry IV Pt II

A determination of disability is a legal concept based on medical evidence. Lawyers and physicians use the same words to mean different things. Impairment, which underlies disability, refers to the symptoms and signs–a painful knee, a clogged artery–in the World Health Organization's [WHO] catalog developed by Professor Philip Wood (1). To the legal profession, it often means the consequence thereof: a "documentation and quantification of reduction of bodily or organ function" (2). By general agreement, the medical profession contributes these data. Again, to the WHO, disability is the functional consequence of impairment (1), and part of that definition is subsumed in the legal concept of impairment itself. The extension, task-specific limitation in performance, is the legal definition (2), and overlaps into WHO's handicap, the social consequence of disability (1). While there are variations in the ways these terms are applied, and different legal systems approach them differently, some unanimity exists. Whether or not a "safety net" is created for those suffering impairments and disabilities, the medical approach addresses the impairment and only secondarily the disability [it is not by coincidence that the initial definition of inflammation referred to pain, redness, swelling and heat, all impairment characteristics and only later added functional loss, the recognition of disability]. How often impairment leads to disability and the latter to handicap [a painful knee may be difficult to walk on–the disability–but the flight of stairs turns it into handicap so that the job cannot be done] needs more studies, especially in areas that have neither codified nor compensated disability, but in most highly developed industrialized nations, the law recognizes inabilities consequent to physical or mental trauma or disease and provides for some type of financial and medical support. In these societies, evidence is crucial, and is provided by the medical profession [in extenso, as not only physicians but other professionals who offer care or diagnosis may be called upon]. But the determination that the injury, insult or illness has led to disability generally devolves upon an administrative law judge or referee or court, based on the evidence provided by the examiner and experts brought in to testify about some special aspects (3). Thus, while patients [i.e., individuals who seek diagnosis and care] expect those they consult for care to obtain for them what they assume they can attain under the law, the results are in the hands of those they have thus consulted only to the extent of giving testimony, serving as evidence, providing facts upon which others rule. Immoderate promises to patients and qualified evidence can lead to results adverse to claimants' desires.

The contretemps arising from the different approaches of law and medicine is starkly dramatized in extreme situations, as discussed in the *New England Journal of Medicine*. One essay (4) addressed the standard of emergency care as it applied to an anencephalic infant. Baby K, whose condition was known beforehand, had difficulty breathing at birth and was mechanically ventilated. As mechanical ventilation served no therapeutic or palliative purpose, the physicians urged the mother to permit its discontinuation; she refused. The case worked its way through the courts. The hospital, its ethics committee, the baby's father, and the guardian appointed by the court believed that such assistance should not be offered. The trial judge focused on antidiscrimination legislation in his opinion that the hospital was obligated to provide care as the mother wished. Nowhere in section 504 of the Rehabilitation Act and the Americans with Disabilities Act was anencephaly exempted from coverage by their provisions, and as a general matter of law, parents have the right to make decisions about medical treatment for their children. The appellate court affirmed this judgment by a split [two to one] decision, by focusing entirely on the single question, did Congress mean to exempt anencephalic infants in respiratory distress [almost a burlesque, if not so serious, of the reasons given by the Mikado for not voiding the death sentence of Koko and his colleagues].

Applicable to our discussion are the "mixed messages and confused roles" that directly address impairment and disability. The court held that the emergency condition was respiratory distress [a disability], not anencephaly [an impairment, if an extreme one], as the hospital [viz. medical profession] had argued. The second contention, that medical treatment outside the prevailing standard of medical care should not be required, found a sympathetic response in the Court, but it was up to Congress, not the courts, to redress such concerns.

The author of the article, a lawyer with public health credentials and expertise, enumerates the misjudgments in his analysis. The major misjudgment, he believes, was the trial judge's, who reduced the question to, "can ventilatory support help an anencephalic infant in respiratory distress" and answered "yes." The discussion of this error is instructive, as similar questions [but not in anencephaly; the problem had never come up in this fashion] have already been answered by Congress and the executive branch [the Baby Doe regulations that recognized limits on care and the role of reasonable medical judgment]. The "law of unintended consequences" once more rears its ugly head: the whole process could have been avoided if the phrase, "consistent with reasonable medical standards" had been inserted among the requirements of the Act. The author recommends, to avoid having appropriate medical care be decided by payers and regulators and a situation in which physicians will do whatever patients want [turning their work into a consumer product], standards must be set and adhered to. But the differences between law and medicine are stark. The physicians really did treat the anencephalic embryo, fetus, and infant as if it were–or was developing to be, or could eventually become–a sentient human being. Their administration of ventilatory aid initially clearly was a humanitarian automatic response, without which the whole problem would never have come about.

Thus, the differences in definitions of impairment and disability in medicine and law, and the lack of clarity to the laiety/patient produced this quixotic problem. In a less charged fashion, the misunderstandings apply to musculoskeletal disability as well. Already backache, vaguely defined musculoskeletal disorders, and the less common specific arthritides have achieved the unenviable distinction of being leading causes for worker's compensation, job absenteeism, and high-priced product liability ascriptions [look at silicone implants, for example, which, thanks to Berkson's fallacy, concentrated a melange of such cases in specialists' offices and led to unproved associations, compensation, and court actions, not to mention the controversies that have driven the rheumatologic profession to sidetaking] (5).

In rheumatology, the responsibilities of the physician are awesome. There are no pulse rates and blood pressures and different types of cardiography; there are no pulmonary function tests; there is no measurement of renal blood flow and urine output, BUN and other laboratory measurements.

Indeed, for many rheumatic disorders, there are few if any reproducible measurements–erythrocyte sedimentation rate is nonspecific, x-rays and their embellishments reflect chiefly late disease [and often cannot correlate with function], and only joint fluid analysis and arthroscopy bid to confirm the clinical impression. Most measurements that are thought to be indispensable reflect Dubos's dictum: The measurable drives out the important. But measurements of some sort are important, as compensation often builds on functional loss. When no obvious physical lesion is present [and sometimes even when there is], deficits can reflect motivation and effort on the part of the patient and skill and emphasis on the part of the examiner (6). For example, physical therapists are interested in gross movements, occupational therapists in finer movements [as by the hand], and rehabilitation nurses are most concerned with the amount of assistance a patient needs and ability for self-care. Thus, their respective assessments differ. Physicians often have others fill in some of the blanks on assessment forms and frequently color their observations by their diagnoses; surgeons, of course, tend to emphasize mechanical restoration. The patient's cooperation in turn devolves in part upon the secondary gain, the desire to cooperate and please, and specific needs. A small loss of range of motion in the hand and fingers may be disastrous to a jeweler, a dentist, a surgeon, a pianist or a keyboard operator, while of little consequence to the stevedore; loss of hip and knee motion impedes the work of the laborer and may not affect the work of the sedentary and professional. Availability of responsive public transportation can minimize the access problem for some city dwellers while need for transport in stock cars can undo the suburbanite and rural individual. Thus, assessment on pretested and validated scales, in addition to the examination and history, and appreciation of these in the psychosocial setting need to be documented by the physician. No adequate measure of stiffness nor objective measure of pain is available.

Another problem arises in diagnostic label, often required in such assessments. Different boundaries to a diagnosis are features of different systems and cultures: fibrositis, fibromyalgia, generalized tendomyopathy, and even psychophysiological musculoskeletal reaction cover overlapping territories, depending on the geographical site of examination, but are not really the same condition. And when it comes to prognosis, they are even more difficult to categorize and verify.

Clearly, a systematic pattern of recording and careful notes and relevant data become all important in the files of the treating physician, and an acceptable and established schema of documentation in the hands of the consultant asked by the litigants or the social system to render an opinion.

An example of the need for scrupulous recording brought this home to me. I was called in to testify in a case of a woman who had used a hair dye after testing herself for local skin allergy but had nevertheless developed a severe toxic reaction, leading to exfoliation of the scalp, absorption of the dye into the circulation, partial bone marrow depression, consequent massive corticosteroid administration, recovery of blood and skin but aseptic necrosis of the hips, surgical replacement of the hips, failure of the replacement, and ultimate wheelchair existence. I was asked only about the possible role of corticosteroids in promoting avascular necrosis of femoral heads. During the course of my testimony, I was asked whether rheumatoid arthritis could promote avascular hip necrosis and whether corticosteroids are sometimes offered as treatment of rheumatoid arthritis, to both of which I answered affirmatively. The woman had more than twenty documented hospitalizations, and from my vantage point, the sequence and ultimate responsibility seemed obvious. The attorney for the defendant company then produced the record of another hospitalization. One New Year's Eve, the woman's pain had become excruciating. Her physician was unavailable, and the doctor covering for him was unknown to the patient and lived some distance away. However, a local practitioner maintained an office on the corner of her block. She found him in, and he suggested that she would be better served by an overnight hospitalization; on New Year's Day or the next day, her own physician could rescue her. She assented, was given narcotic analgesia overnight, and transferred to her own doctor's outpatient care the next day. But the local doctor signed her out on the discharge sheet as having rheumatoid arthritis. This one reference to this disease led to a verdict for the defendant, despite the judge's charge to the jury to find for the plaintiff. When interviewed later, the local physician proved not to realize that rheumatoid arthritis was a specific diagnosis with specific connotations. To him, all joint pains were rheumatoid arthritis.

However, the courts have held that it is not required that all of the medical evidence and testimony point consistently toward the conclusion reached by the medical expert called in to testify as to causation, and in the case cited, that dictum was ignored by the jury, as will sometimes happen. Probably that resulted from another precedent in the courts, that medical testimony as to causation remains valid even if other conclusions are possible. So it behooves the examiner to document in as much detail as possible the presentation of the disorder, a chronological sequence, and confirmatory evidence to support the clinical construct.

As a witness, the physician should also be as knowledgeable about the condition under discussion to validate the diagnosis and attribution. The physician is an advocate for the truth, not for the plaintiff or defendant, and the "hired gun" will generally be exposed in court and discredited. That does not mean, however, that the opinion must necessarily conform to textbook descriptions. As an example, anecdotal reports of ankylosing spondylitis and reactive arthropathies developing after trauma appear in medical journals and court records. Yet, given a disease of unknown etiology [even if pathogenesis has become clearer], substantiation of a cause and effect–or better, a precipitation or aggravation and effect–relationship is more difficult. There are rationales for this sequence, however, although in the days before HLA-B27 and other genetic factors were recognized, the Ontario Workmen's [sic] Compensation Board held that no relationship existed between trauma and subsequent development or flare of ankylosing spondylitis (7). This decision should not today remain unchallenged. Conversely, while depression, sleep disturbances, and desire for compensation for injury are legitimate responses to traumatic events, and are associated with fibromyalgic symptoms, the case for post-traumatic fibromyalgia is weaker, perhaps chiefly because of the lack of objectification.

Another area of importance is prognosis. The rheumatic diseases are often difficult to prove; they are even more difficult to prognosticate. Yet physicians are constantly asked to address this question, and few clues point to the course a given illness will take in a given individual. Some data exist for groups, but practically none for the individual (8). Thus, the notable associations of educational level with course of rheumatoid arthritis, the correlations with the number of joints involved at the initial appraisal, and similar epidemiologic studies [of Pincus and Callahan and of Hadler and of Hochberg, and others] permit an approximation to be made, but obviously many with similar features follow a different pathway (9). But at least there has been some improvement in outlook since David Hawkins uttered his memorable pairing: While neurology deals with the diagnosis of untreatable disease, rheumatology deals with the treatment of untreatable disease (10). "I don't know" remains an acceptable answer, because formulas have been developed that permit the courts to decide when the appropriate complete data are forthcoming.

REFERENCES

1. Wood FHN, Badley EM: People with Disabilities-Toward Acquiring Information Which Reflects More Sensitively Their Problems and Needs. World Rehabilitation Fund, New York, 1980.

2. Goldstein G: Evaluation of musculoskeletal impairment and function. Medicolegal Consequences of Trauma. Edited by WH Simon, GE Ehrlich. Marcel Dekker, New York, 1993, pp. 29-44.

3. Bond TR: Causation concepts in Workers' Compensation Law: The expanding scope of compensable injuries. Medicolegal Consequences of Trauma. Edited by WH Simon, GE Ehrlich. Marcel Dekker, New York, 1993, 1-28.

4. Annas GJ: Asking the courts to set the standard of emergency care-the case of Baby K. NEJMed 330:1542-1545, 1994.

5. Hadler N: Can trauma "activate" (aggravate) arthritis? Medicolegal Consequences of Trauma. Edited by WH Simon, GE Ehrlich. Marcel Dekker, New York, 1993, 255-294.

6. Ehrlich GE: Arthritis and its problems. Clin Rheum 7:305-320, 1981.

7. Simon WH, Steinberg ME, Ehrlich GE: Long-term consequences of joint injury: avascular necrosis and posttraumatic arthritis. Medicolegal Consequences of Trauma. Edited by WH Simon, GE Ehrlich. Marcel Dekker, New York, 1993, 155-192.

8. Fries JF, Ehrlich GE: Prognosis. The Charles Press, Brady Company, Prentice Hall, Bowie, MD, 1981.

9. Callahan LF, Pincus T: Formal educational level as a significant marker of clinical status in rheumatoid arthritis. Arthr Rheum, 31:1346-1357, 1988.

10. Ehrlich GE: Factors affecting the choice of drug and response to treatment. Drug Therapy in Rheumatology. Edited by SH Roth, PSG, Littleton, MA, 1985, 1-37.

The Cost of Long Term Disability Due to Fibromyalgia, Chronic Fatigue Syndrome and Repetitive Strain Injury: The Private Insurance Perspective

Robert S. Cameron

SUMMARY. Objectives: To examine current group long term disability claims due to chronic fatigue syndrome, fibromyalgia and repetitive strain injury and develop expected claims costs.

Methods: We reviewed a sample of active disability claims to determine diagnoses and costs and the results were projected over the total caseload and the industry as a whole.

Results: Chronic fatigue syndrome represented 78 claims producing monthly payments of $109,000. Fibromyalgia represented 224 claims producing monthly payments of $182,000. Repetitive strain injury represented 149 claims producing monthly payments of $121,000. Similar costs would total over $100 million annually across the industry.

Conclusions: Long term disability caused by these conditions results in very significant claims payments by the group insurance industry in Canada.

Robert S. Cameron, MD, DLIM, is Medical Director, Employee Benefits Division, London Life Insurance Company and Occupational Health Medical Consultant, Canada Post Corporation, Central Division.

Address correspondence to: Dr. R. S. Cameron, 116 Pitcarnie Road, London, Ontario, Canada N6G 4N4.

[Haworth co-indexing entry note]: "The Cost of Long Term Disability Due to Fibromyalgia, Chronic Fatigue Syndrome and Repetitive Strain Injury: The Private Insurance Perspective." Cameron, Robert S. Co-published simultaneously in the *Journal of Musculoskeletal Pain* (The Haworth Medical Press, an imprint of The Haworth Press, Inc.) Vol. 3, No. 2, 1995, pp. 169-172; and: *Fibromyalgia, Chronic Fatigue Syndrome, and Repetitive Strain Injury: Current Concepts in Diagnosis, Management, Disability, and Health Economics* (ed: Andrew Chalmers et al.) The Haworth Press, an imprint of The Haworth Press, Inc., 1995, pp. 169-172. Multiple copies of this article/chapter may be purchased from The Haworth Document Delivery Center [1-800-3-HAWORTH; 9:00 a.m. - 5:00 p.m. (EST)].

© 1995 by The Haworth Press, Inc. All rights reserved.

169

KEYWORDS. Disability, fibromyalgia, chronic fatigue syndrome, repetitive strain injury

Chronic fatigue syndrome [CFS], fibromyalgia and repetitive strain injury [RSI] are significant causes of long term disability in Canada. They present a major challenge for private disability insurers due to their highly subjective natures, uncertain durations and substantial costs. We examined the current experience of London Life Insurance Company, a large Canadian life insurance company with significant business in the group long term disability market. The experience at London Life was used to develop projected costs for the group long term disability industry as a whole.

METHODS

Long term disability claims at London Life can be categorized by multiple characteristics, one being the cause code, which indicates the primary condition producing the disability. We reviewed a representative sample of active group long term disability claims with cause codes representing musculoskeletal disorders. Claims with the specific diagnoses of fibromyalgia or RSI underwent further analysis and the results were extrapolated over London Life's full caseload of approximately 8,000 claims.

London Life uses a unique cause code for the diagnoses of CFS, therefore we were able to analyze all active group long term disability claims where CFS was the primary condition producing the disability.

We projected the impact of these conditions on the private group insurance industry at large by assuming similar prevalences to those found at London Life and multiplying by a factor determined by London Life's share of the group long term disability market.

RESULTS

Fibromyalgia was found in 11.2% of the musculoskeletal claims reviewed, representing 2.8% of all group long term disability claims. This prevalence translates to 224 active claims. The average claim payment was $813 per month resulting in total claims payments of $182,115 per month. On an annualized basis, these amounts would represent an average claim payment of $9,754 and total claims payments of $2,185,344. The large majority also received Canada Pension disability benefits, which resulted in a reduction in the insurance benefit payable.

Repetitive strain injury was found in 7.6% of the musculoskeletal claims reviewed, representing 1.9% of all group long term disability claims. This prevalence translates to 149 active claims. The average claim payment was $815 per month resulting in total claims payments of $121,435 per month. On an annualized basis, these amounts would represent an average claim payment of $9,781 and total claims payments of $1,457,220. The large majority also received other disability benefits, which resulted in a reduction in the insurance benefit payable.

Chronic fatigue syndrome was the primary diagnosis in 78 claims, representing 1% of all group long term disability claims. The average claim payment was $1,398 per month resulting in total claims payments of $109,018 per month. On an annualized basis, these amounts would represent an average claim payment of $16,722 and total claims payments of $1,308,216.

Recent figures for New Sales Revenue and Total Revenue indicate that London Life has almost 5% of the group long term disability insurance market in Canada. Figures are not available specifically for group long term disability claims payments, but would be expected to be very similar. Using this market share and generalizing the prevalences found at London Life, it could be expected that group long term disability insurers in Canada will pay out approximately $46 million for fibromyalgia claims, $30 million for RSI claims, and $27 million for CFS claims in 1994.

DISCUSSION

The group long term disability insurance market in Canada is highly competitive, with low profit margins typically well under 10%. In this environment, the pressure to control disability claims costs is significant and many insurers are actively pursuing the means to do so. Improving claims adjudication and reducing claim duration are the most effective methods to achieve such control, and opportunities to do so are significant with claims due to CFS, fibromyalgia, and repetitive strain injury. Reliable and objective methods for assessment of severity would help improve the quality of claims adjudication and expedite the prompt approval of qualifying claims. Development of treatment programs which can effectively restore functional capacity would aid insurers in reducing claim duration. Most insurers are quite agreeable to privately funding such programs if they can be provided in a cost effective manner.

CONCLUSION

Long term disability caused by CFS, fibromyalgia, and RSI results in very significant claims payments by group long term disability insurance carriers in Canada. The magnitude of these costs should motivate private insurers to participate in the advancement of the understanding of these conditions, particularly in the areas of assessment of severity and treatment to restore functional capacity.

Index

© 1995 by The Haworth Press, Inc. All rights reserved.

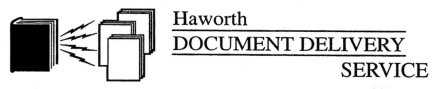

Haworth
DOCUMENT DELIVERY
SERVICE

This new service provides a single-article order form for any article from a Haworth journal.

- *Time Saving:* No running around from library to library to find a specific article.
- *Cost Effective:* All costs are kept down to a minimum.
- *Fast Delivery:* Choose from several options, including same-day FAX.
- *No Copyright Hassles:* You will be supplied by the original publisher.
- *Easy Payment:* Choose from several easy payment methods.

Open Accounts Welcome for . . .
- Library Interlibrary Loan Departments
- Library Network/Consortia Wishing to Provide Single-Article Services
- Indexing/Abstracting Services with Single Article Provision Services
- Document Provision Brokers and Freelance Information Service Providers

MAIL or *FAX* THIS ENTIRE ORDER FORM TO:

Haworth Document Delivery Service
The Haworth Press, Inc.
10 Alice Street
Binghamton, NY 13904-1580

or **FAX:** (607) 722-6362
or **CALL:** 1-800-3-HAWORTH
(1-800-342-9678; 9am-5pm EST)

PLEASE SEND ME PHOTOCOPIES OF THE FOLLOWING SINGLE ARTICLES:

1) Journal Title: _____

    Vol/Issue/Year:_____Starting & Ending Pages:_____

Article Title:_____

2) Journal Title: _____

    Vol/Issue/Year:_____Starting & Ending Pages:_____

Article Title:_____

3) Journal Title: _____

    Vol/Issue/Year:_____Starting & Ending Pages:_____

Article Title:_____

4) Journal Title: _____

    Vol/Issue/Year:_____Starting & Ending Pages:_____

Article Title:_____

(See other side for Costs and Payment Information)

COSTS: Please figure your cost to order quality copies of an article.

1. Set-up charge per article: $8.00
     ($8.00 × number of separate articles) _____

2. Photocopying charge for each article:

     1-10 pages: $1.00 _____

     11-19 pages: $3.00 _____

     20-29 pages: $5.00 _____

     30+ pages: $2.00/10 pages _____

3. Flexicover (optional): $2.00/article _____
4. Postage & Handling: US: $1.00 for the first article/
          $.50 each additional article _____

     Federal Express: $25.00 _____

     Outside US: $2.00 for first article/
          $.50 each additional article _____

5. Same-day FAX service: $.35 per page _____

                    GRAND TOTAL: _____

METHOD OF PAYMENT: (please check one)
❏ Check enclosed   ❏ Please ship and bill. PO # _____
               (sorry we can ship and bill to bookstores only! All others must pre-pay)
❏ Charge to my credit card: ❏ Visa; ❏ MasterCard; ❏ American Express;

Account Number:_____ Expiration date:_____

Signature: ✗_____

Name: _____ Institution: _____

Address: _____

          _____

City: _____ State:_____ Zip:_____

Phone Number: _____ FAX Number: _____

MAIL or *FAX* THIS ENTIRE ORDER FORM TO:

Haworth Document Delivery Service
The Haworth Press, Inc.
10 Alice Street
Binghamton, NY 13904-1580

or FAX: (607) 722-6362
or CALL: 1-800-3-HAWORTH
(1-800-342-9678; 9am-5pm EST)